The Purpose of this Book

Every year thousands of people including doctors, medical students, paramedics, nurses, nursing students, and others involved in the care and treatment of cardiac patients, get introduced to the world of reading electrocardiograms (ECGs or EKGs).

This skill is fundamental to understanding if a patient is having a problem with the rhythm of their heart, has an electrolyte problem, is receiving too much of a given medication, experiencing an infection or inflammation of the heart, has too much fluid around the heart, or are experiencing a myocardial infarction.

While reading an electrocardiogram may seem daunting at first, this book was designed from my lectures used to train students, interns, residents and fellows, on how to read an electrocardiogram. Rather than memorizing facts, this book will walk you through the steps of how to read electrocardiograms from beginning to end using the same approach used by Cardiologists like myself.

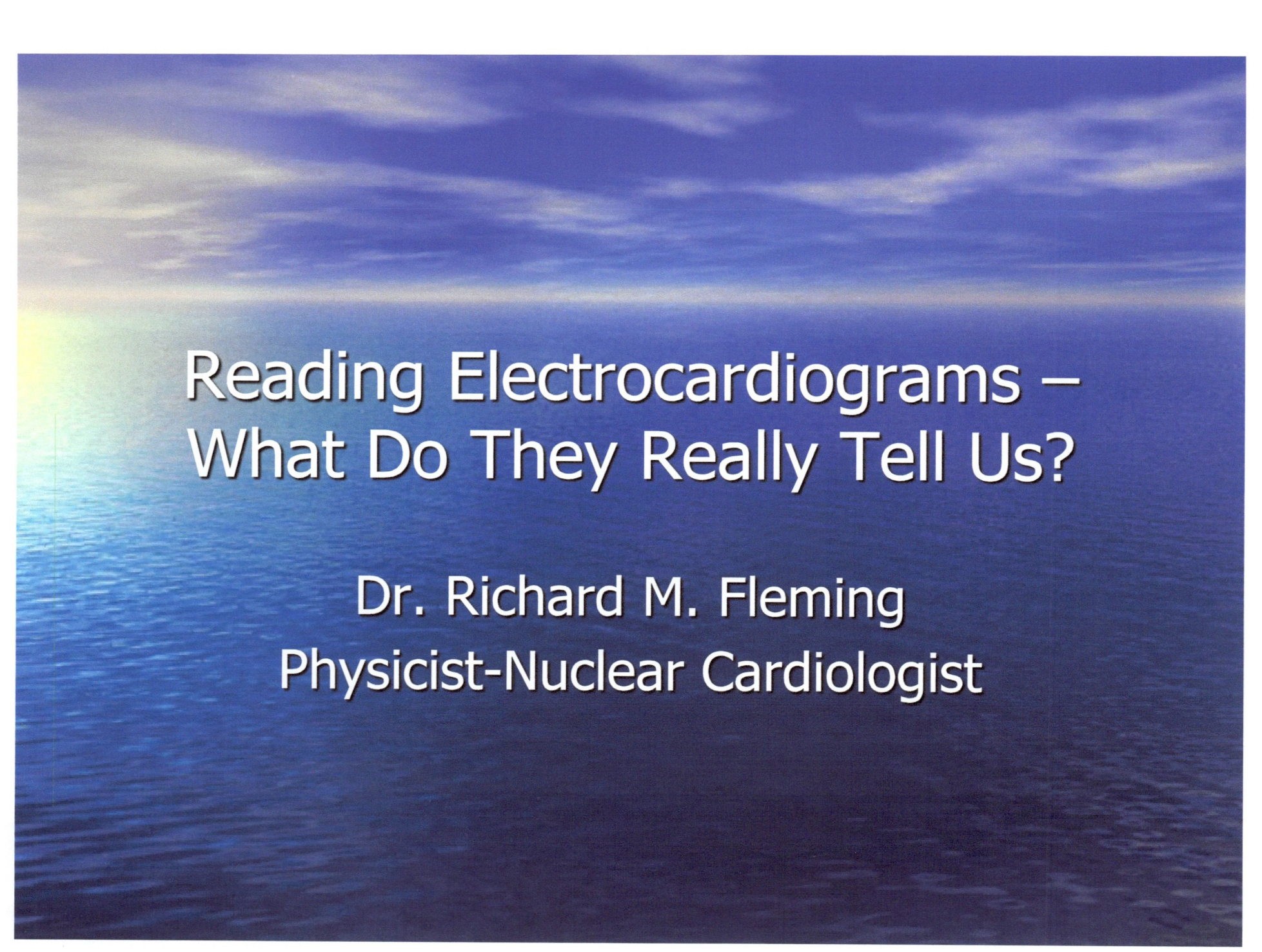

Unfortunately most people have negative (cathode) memories of understanding electricity.

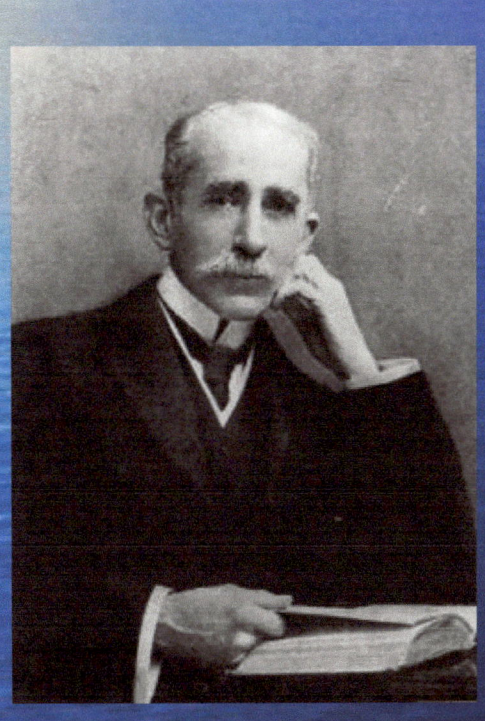

Sir John Ambrose Fleming
Patented the Vacuum Diode
(Converts AC to DC)

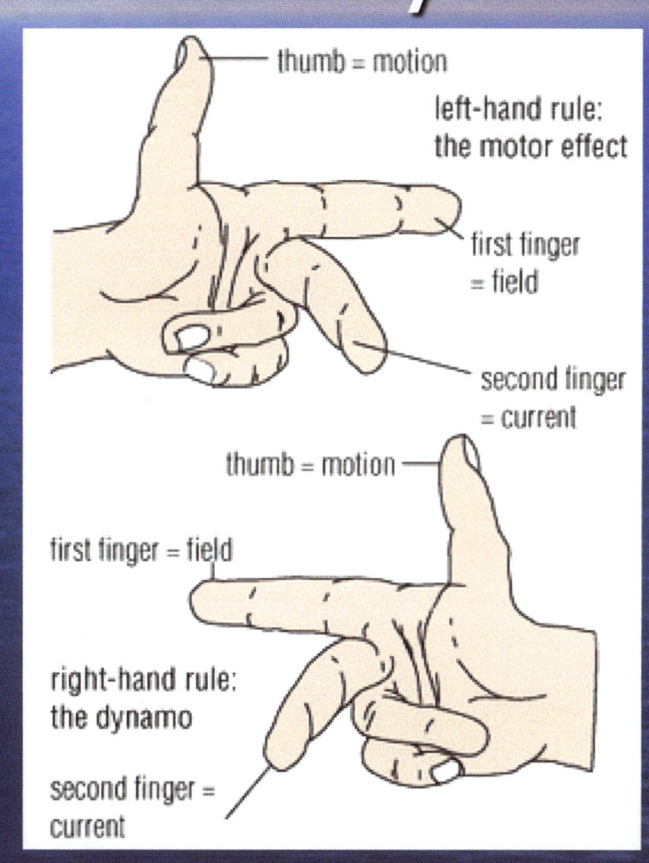

We are looking at electrical systems including: Capacitors (hold charge applied) and Cells (generate electric current).

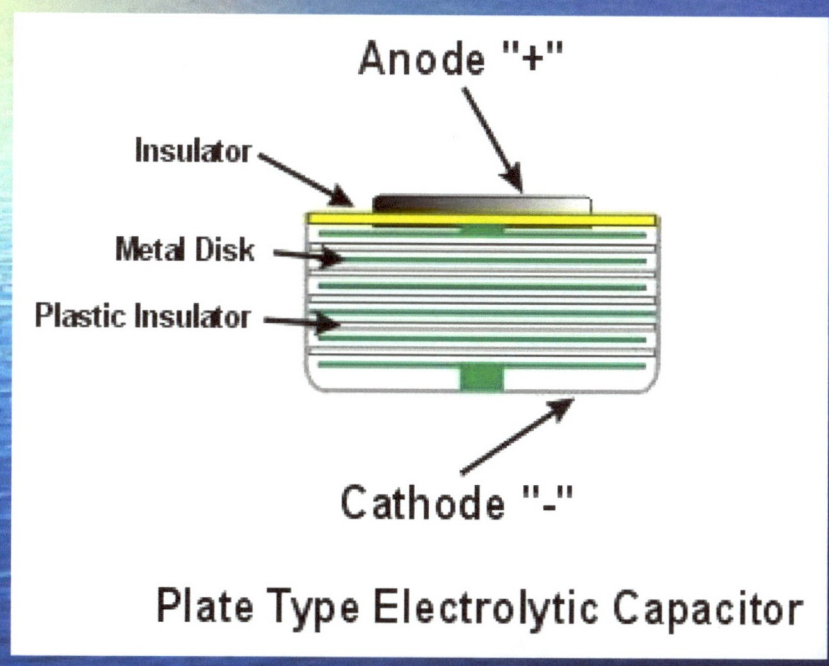

Plate Type Electrolytic Capacitor

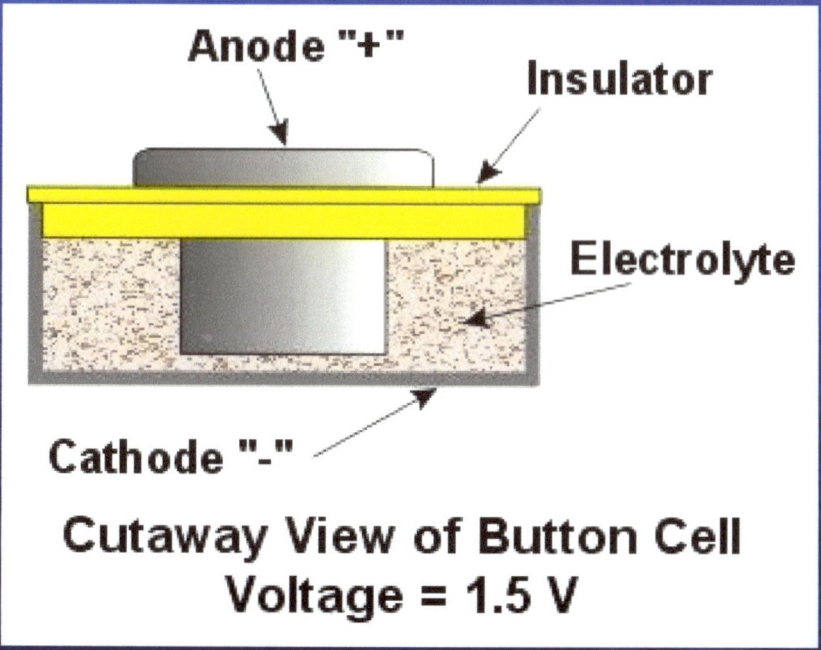

Cutaway View of Button Cell
Voltage = 1.5 V

Capacitors hold electric charge applied to them for discharge later.
Man made cells generate current: electrolyte dissolves cathode.
Batteries are a series of cells joined together.

Used when the Native System Fails: Pacemakers & AICDs (Internally Placed Capacitors and Bateries).

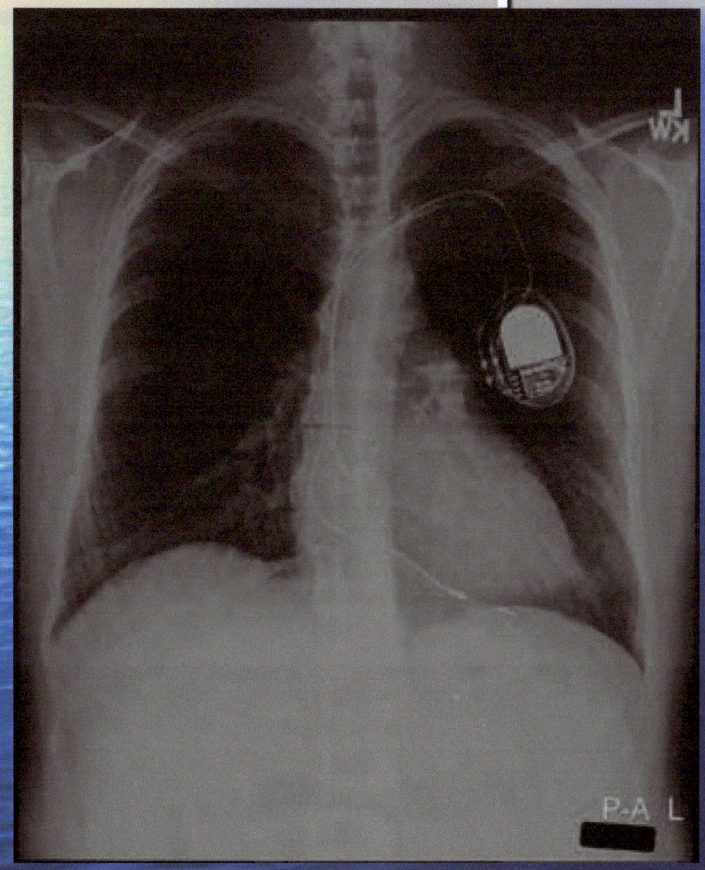
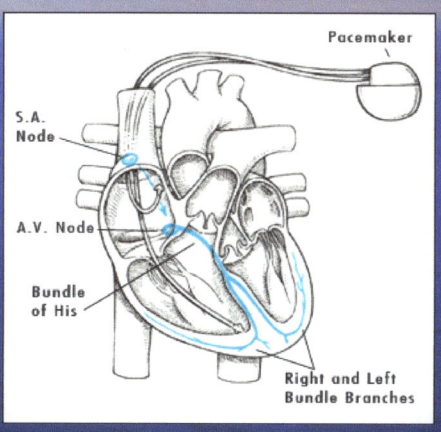
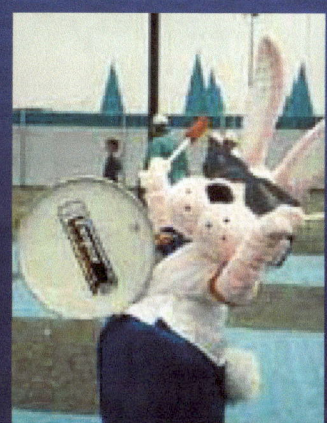

John Hopps, an Electrical Engineer at Univ of Manitoba in 1941, First pacemaker 1950.

The limitations of man made batteries (series of cells) are not biological and therefore cannot regenerate themselves. The more current they discharge, the shorter their life.

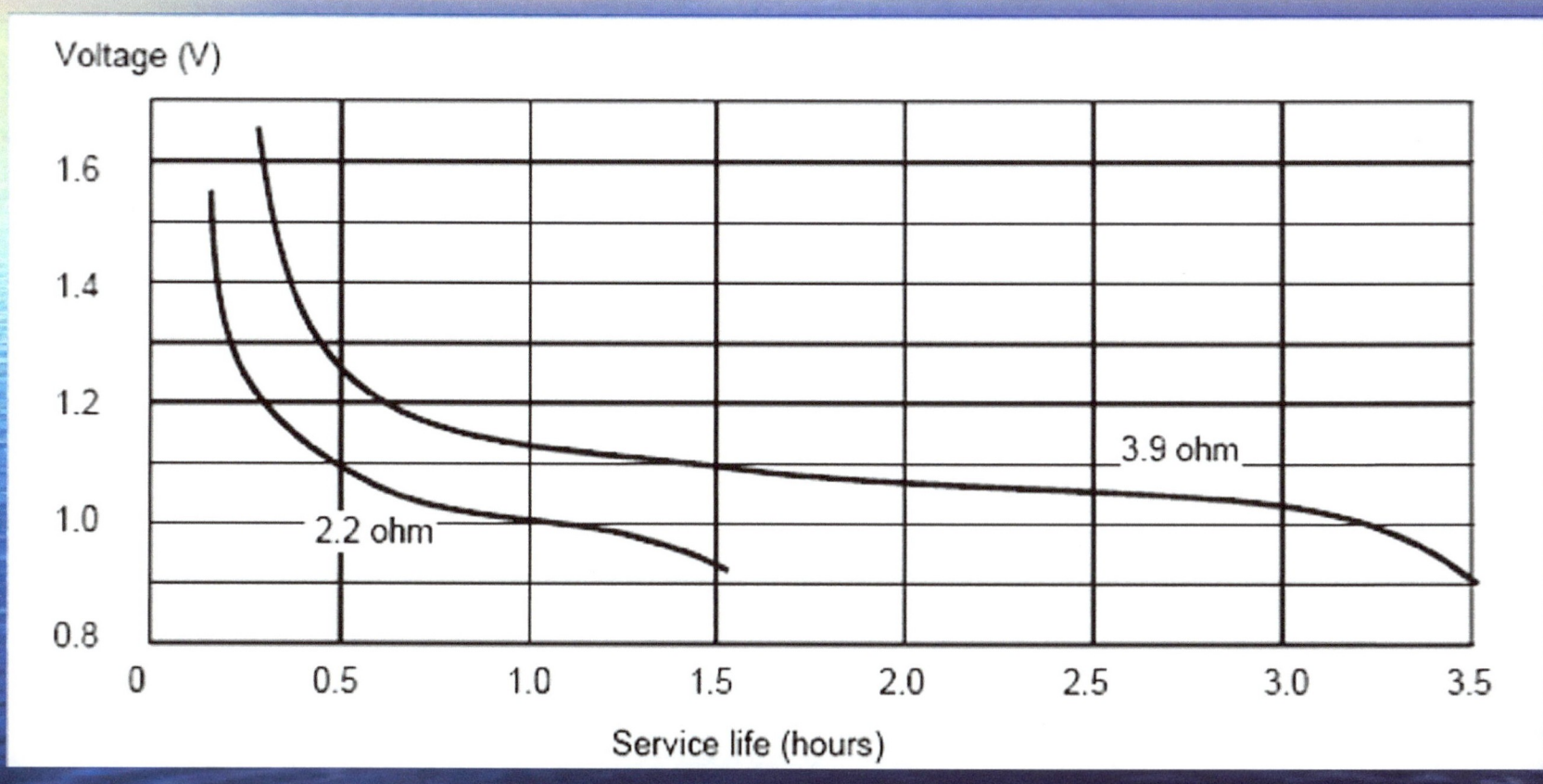

In Contrast Cardiac Tissue:
Both Capacitors (hold charge applied) and Cells (generate electric current).

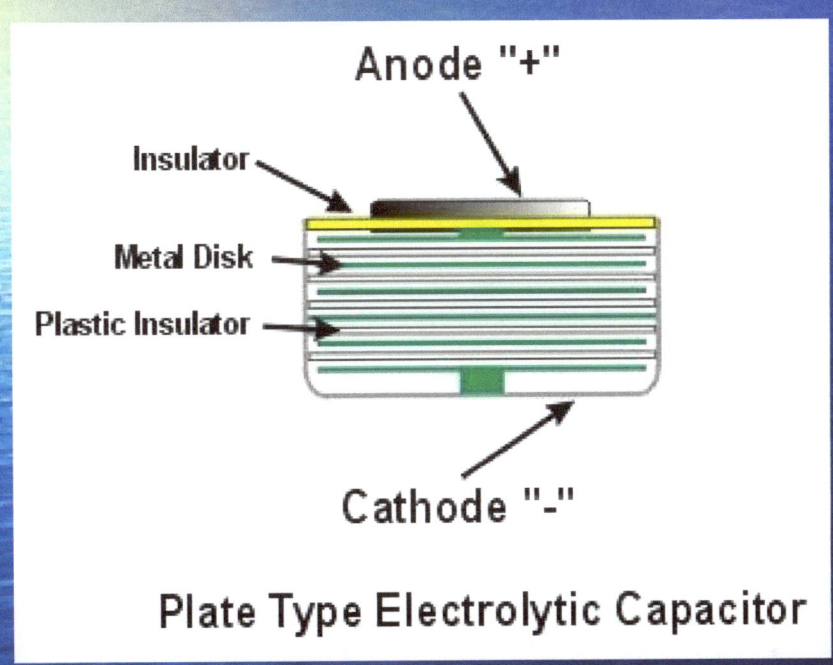

Plate Type Electrolytic Capacitor

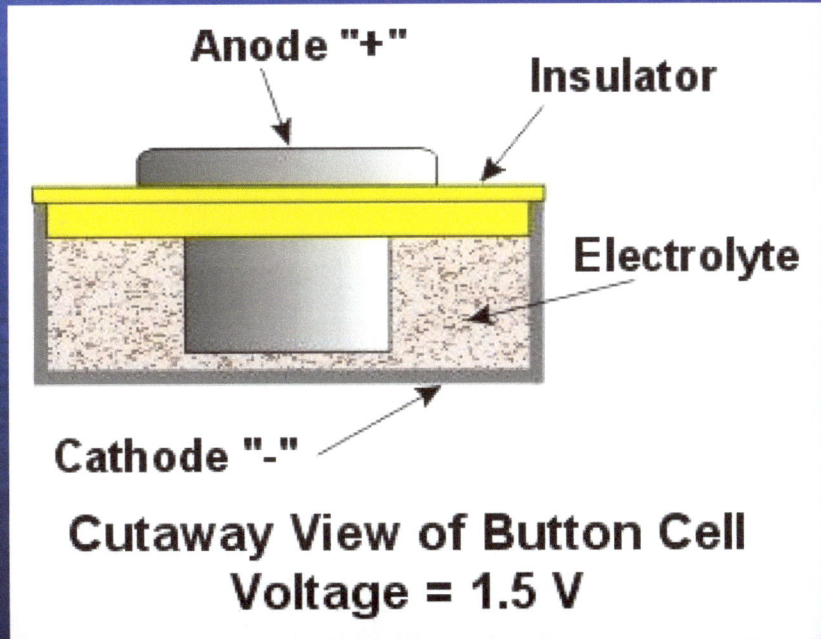

Cutaway View of Button Cell
Voltage = 1.5 V

Capacitors hold electric charge applied to them for discharge later.
Man made cells generate current: electrolyte dissolves cathode.
Batteries are a series of cells joined together.

This is accomplished via energy (mitochondria) expenditure to maintain an in-balance of electrolytes (cathode inside, anode outside of cell).

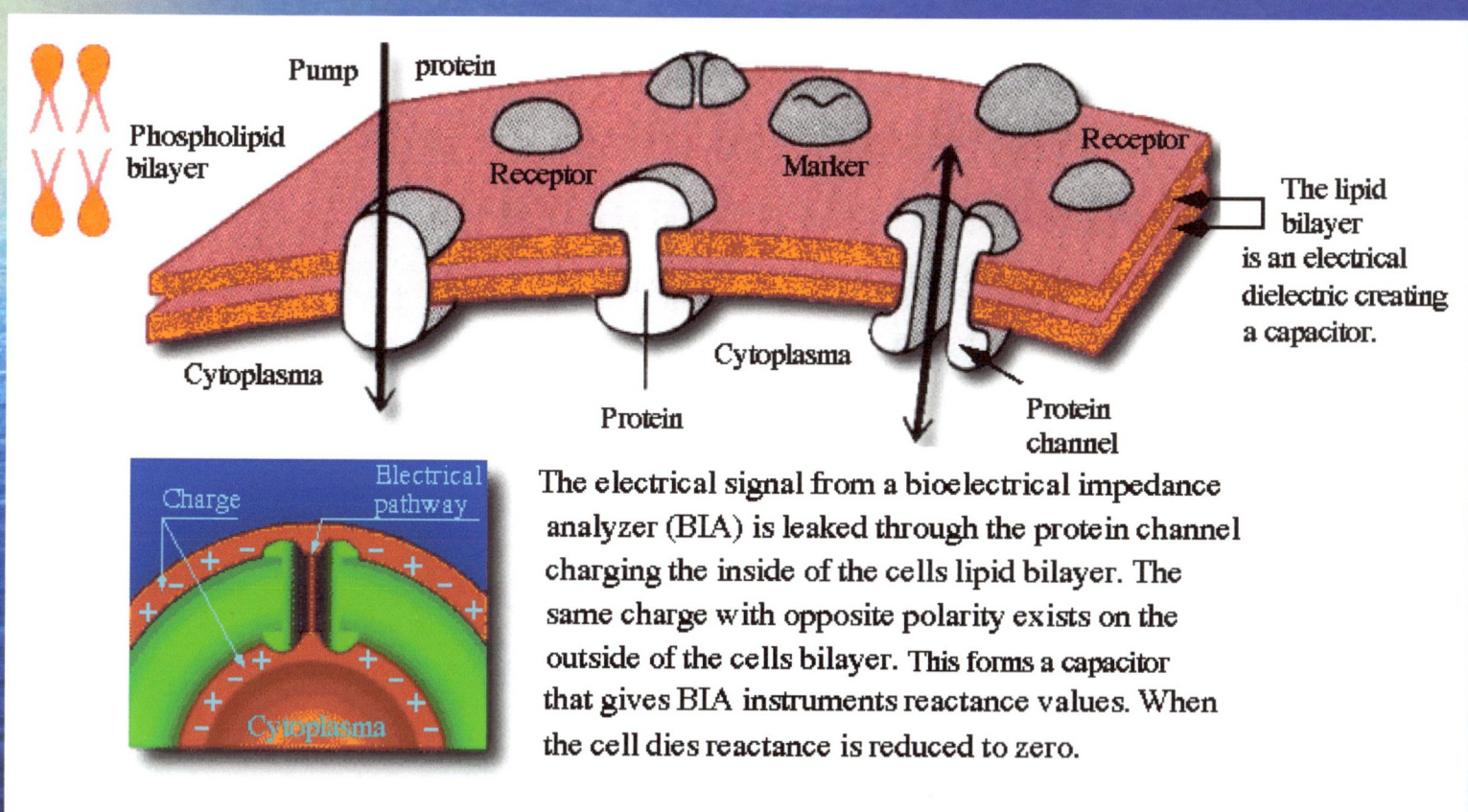

The electrical signal from a bioelectrical impedance analyzer (BIA) is leaked through the protein channel charging the inside of the cells lipid bilayer. The same charge with opposite polarity exists on the outside of the cells bilayer. This forms a capacitor that gives BIA instruments reactance values. When the cell dies reactance is reduced to zero.

Movement of Ions Across Cell Membranes Generate a Current, which is continued as long as the cell is alive and mitochondria are generating energy to maintain electrochemical gradient across cell membrane.

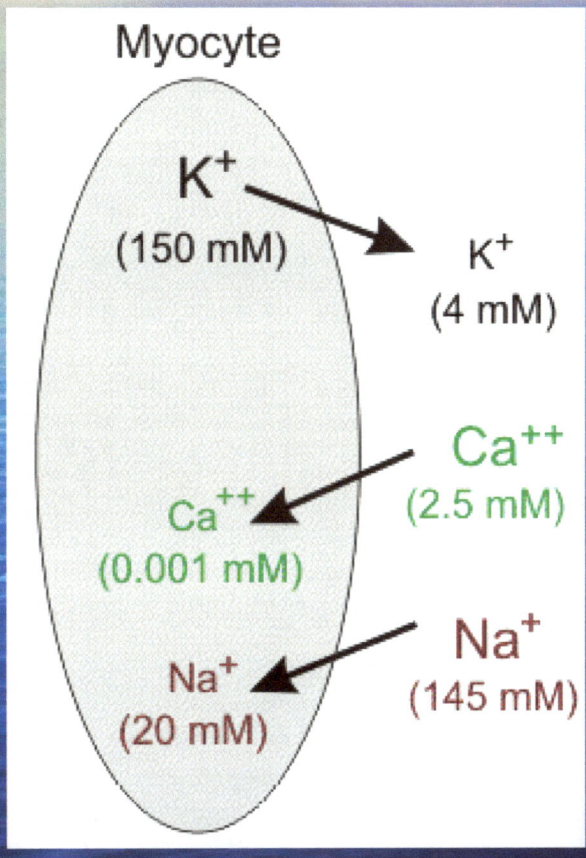

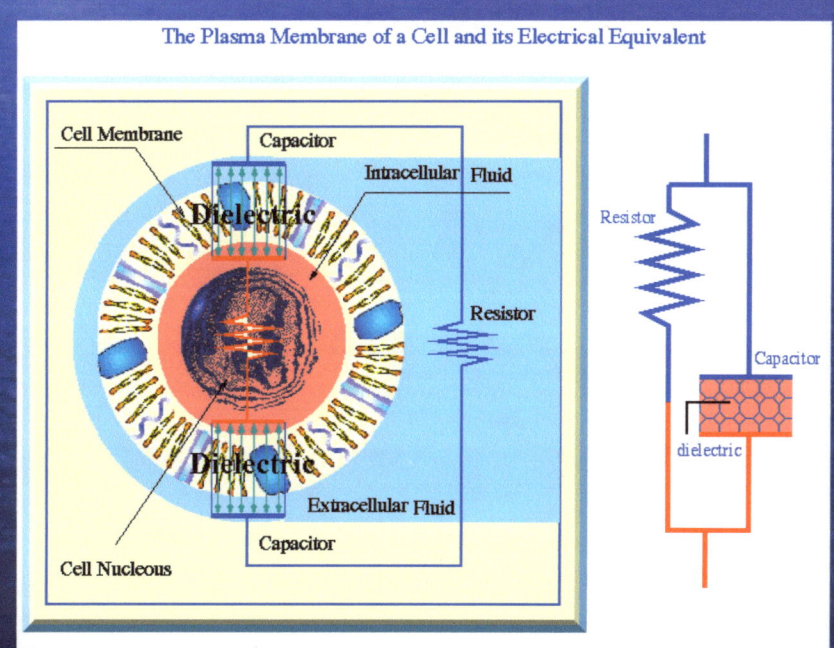

The outer boundary of the cell is a plasma membrane of phospholipid molecules which become a dielectric to form an electrical capacitor when a radio frequency signal is introduced to the cells environment.

Electrical capacitor in PARALLEL with a resistor. Capacitance is analogous to intracellular volume and resistance is analogous to extracellular volume.

Automaticity: SA & AV node Pacemaker & Action Potential.

- The Action Potential (AP) results from:
  - Decreased outward flux of K+
  - Unchanged inward movement of Na+
  - Slow inward leak of Ca++

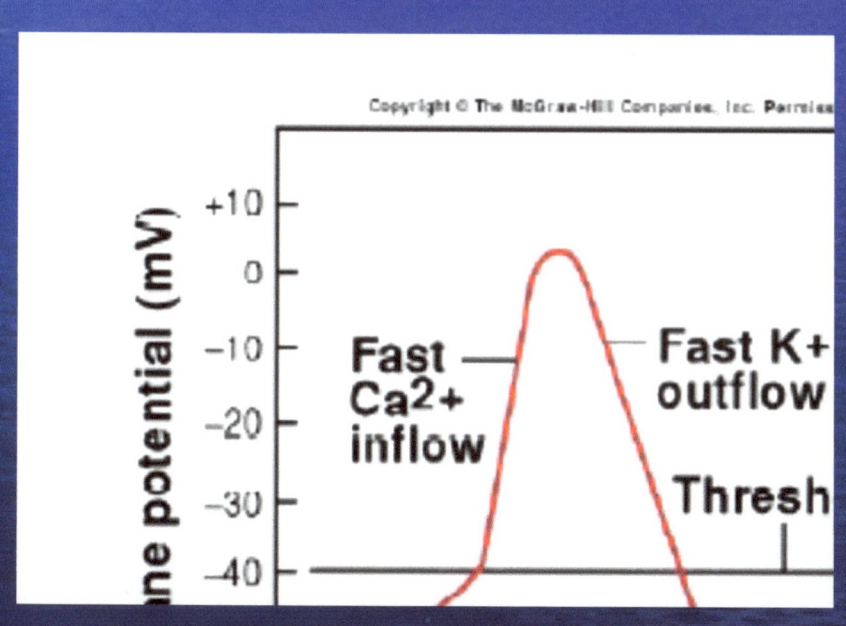

Action Potential of Bundle of His & Myocardium.

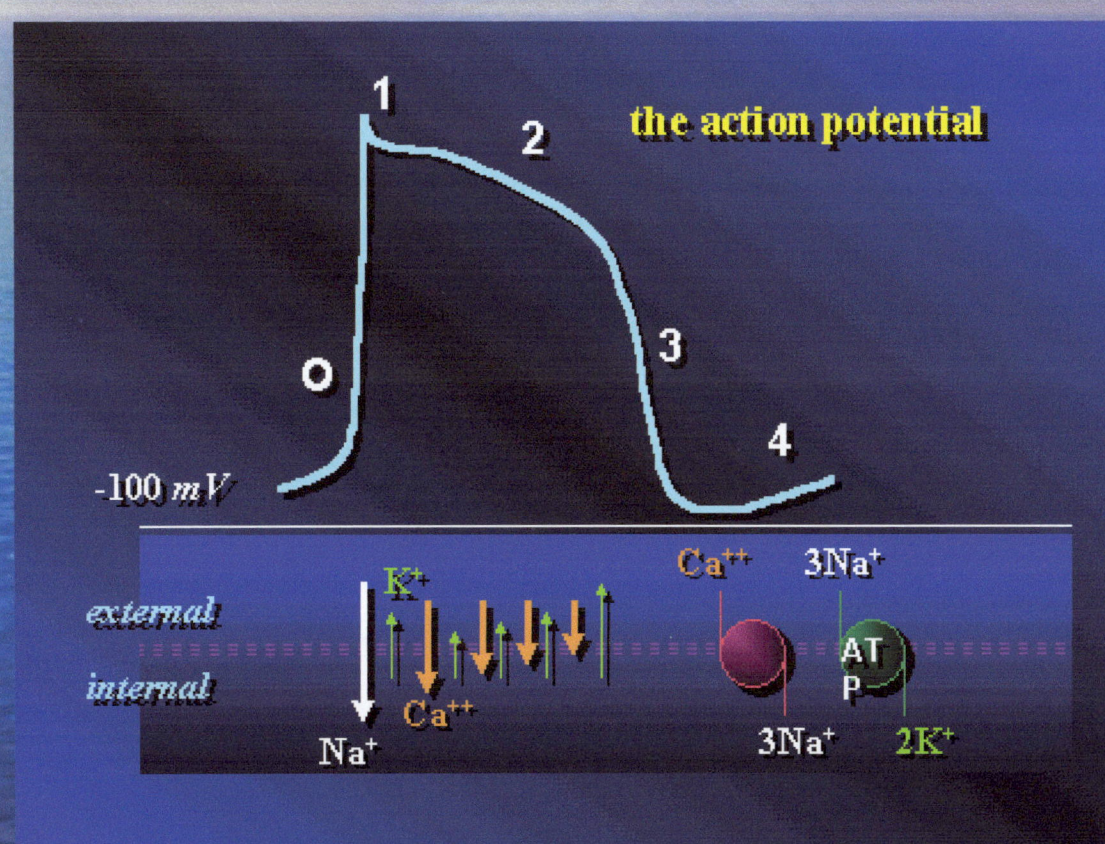

Subsequently the Cells of our Bodies form a Series of Capacitors, Insulators and Resistance - which can be measured.

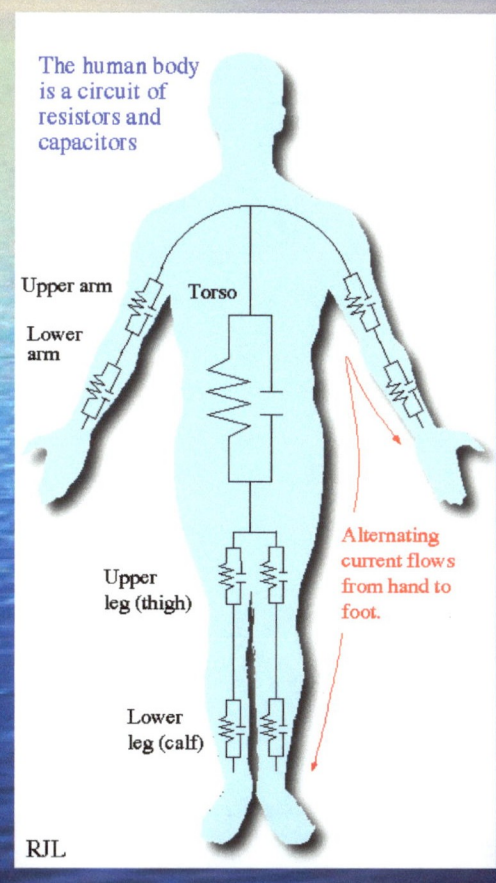

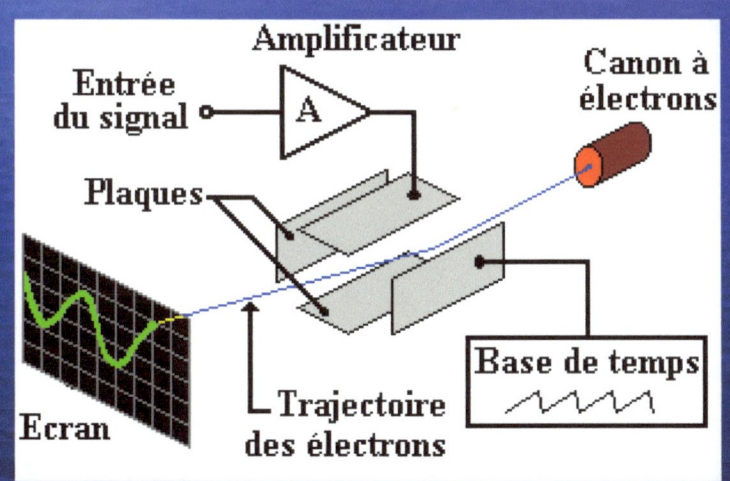

When electrons (depolarization of cardiac cells) moves towards the positive pole of a lead, the oscilloscope signal deflects upwards. When the depolarization moves away from the positive pole of a lead, the deflection is downwards.

Rules of Depolarizataion.
Why the ECG squiggles go up & down.

When electrons (depolarization of cardiac cells) moves towards the positive pole of a lead, the oscilloscope signal deflects upwards.

When the depolarization moves away from the positive pole of a lead, the deflection is downwards.

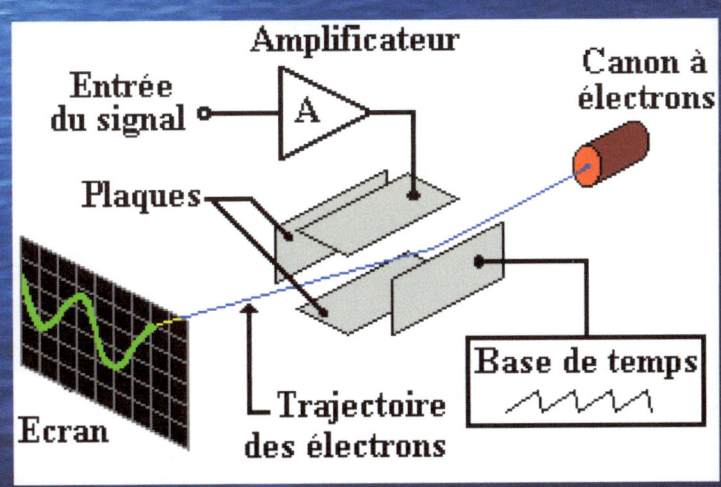

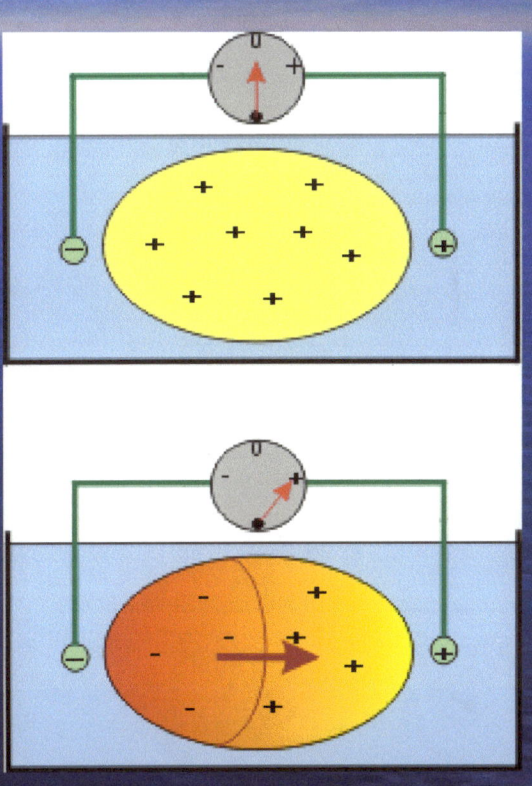

So How do we understand this Conduction System of the Heart, which is a Series of (Usually) Well Connected Electrical Pathways.

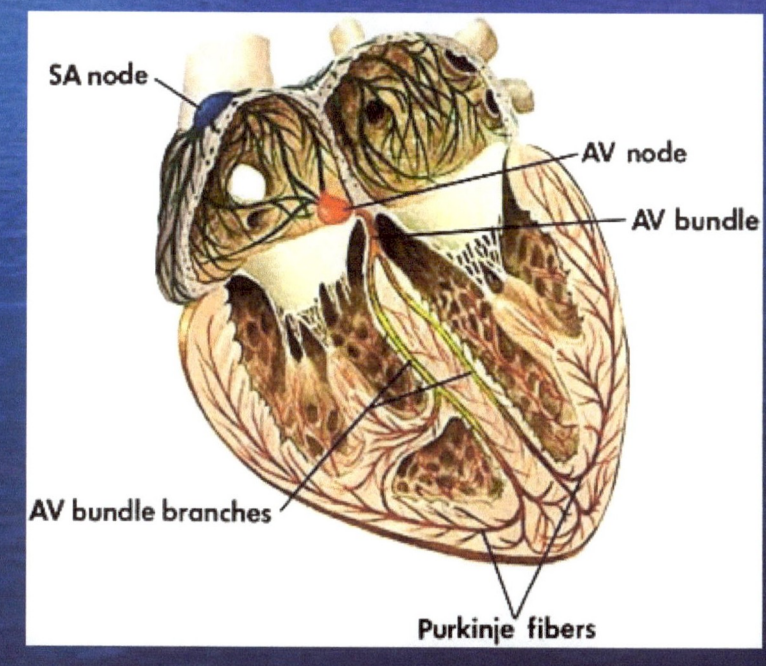

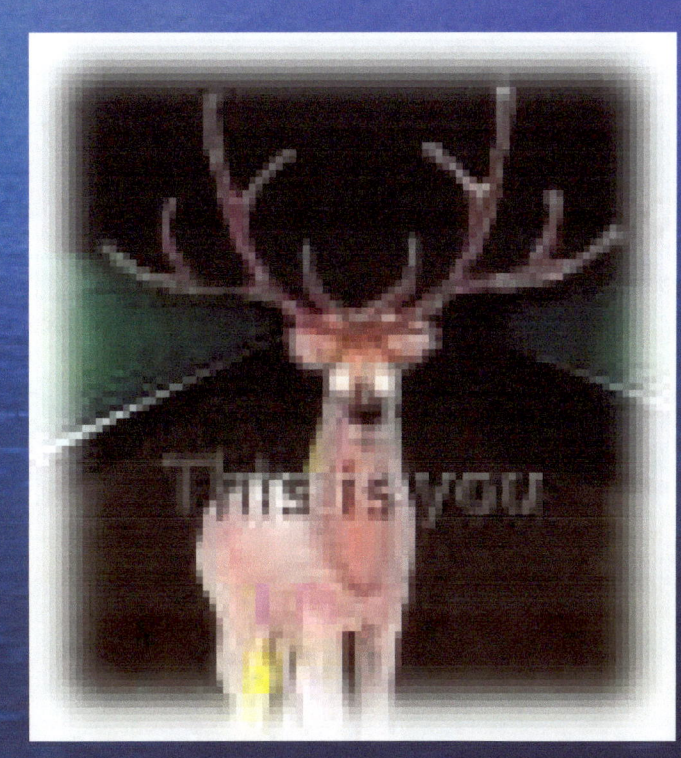

The First Electrocardiograms.

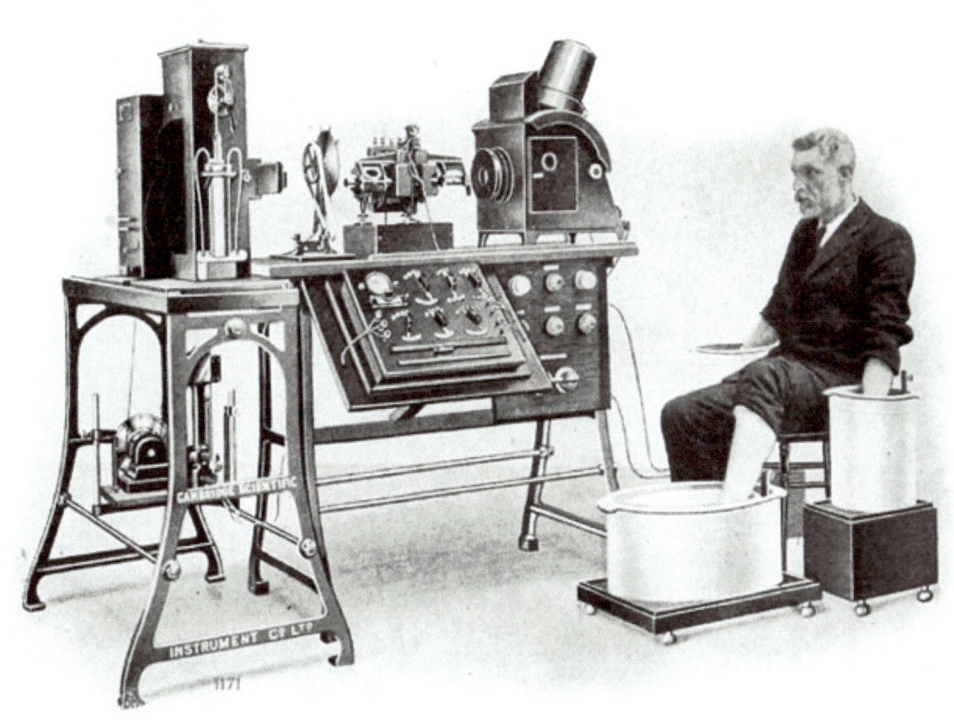

Photograph of a Complete Electrocardiograph, Showing the Manner in which the Electrodes are Attached to the Patient, In this Case the Hands and One Foot Being Immersed in Jars of Salt Solution

Different Leads Given Different Angles/Views of Where the Electrical Activity is Coming from and Going To.

Lead I: Negative RA, Positive LA.
Lead II: Negative RA, Positive LL.
Lead III: Negative LA, Positive LL.

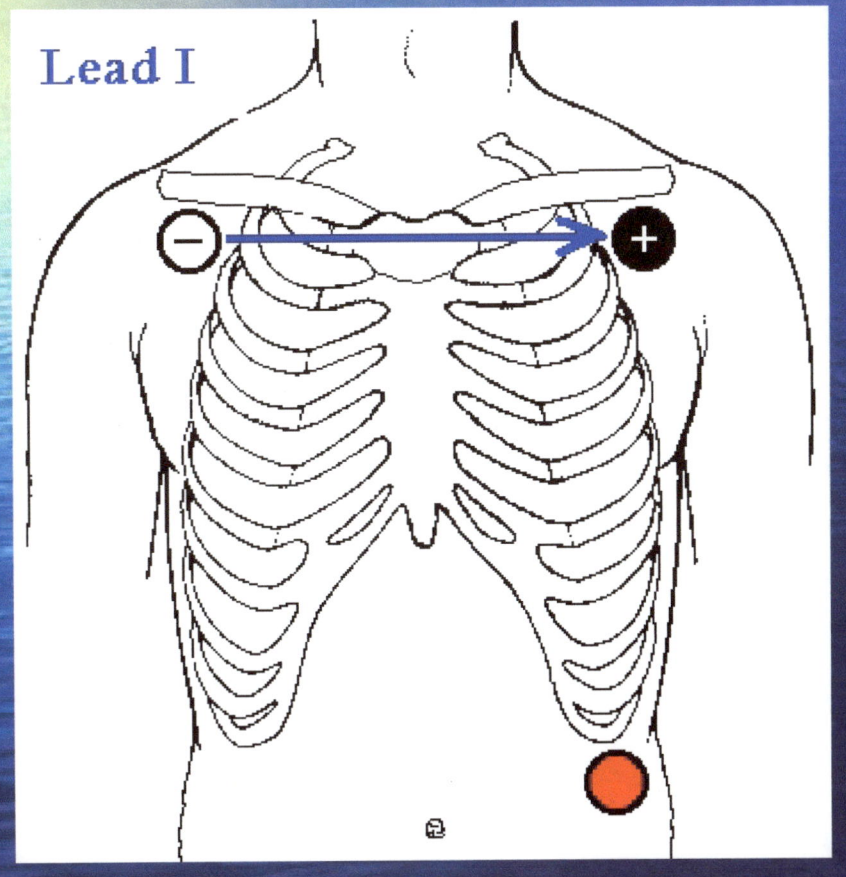
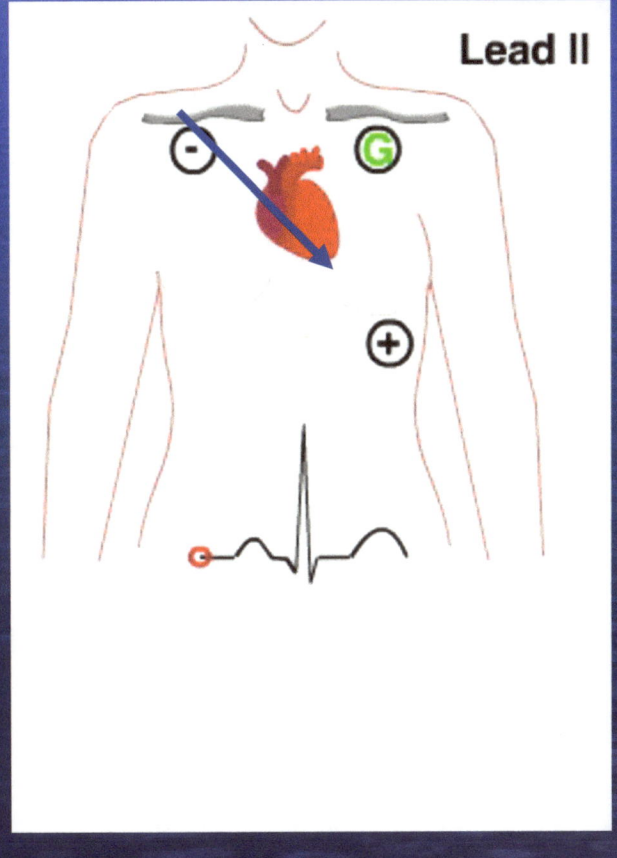

Einthovan's Triangle: Standard Limb Leads.

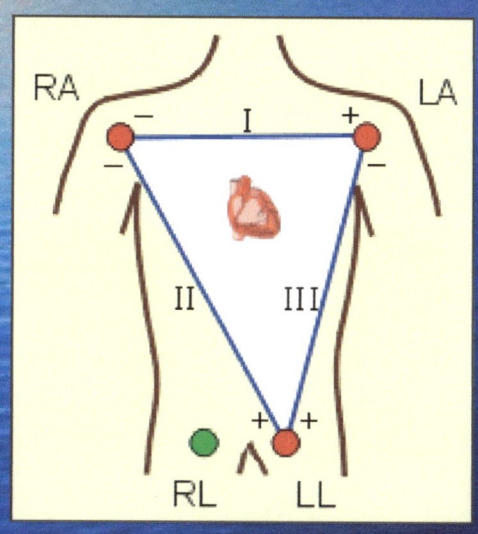
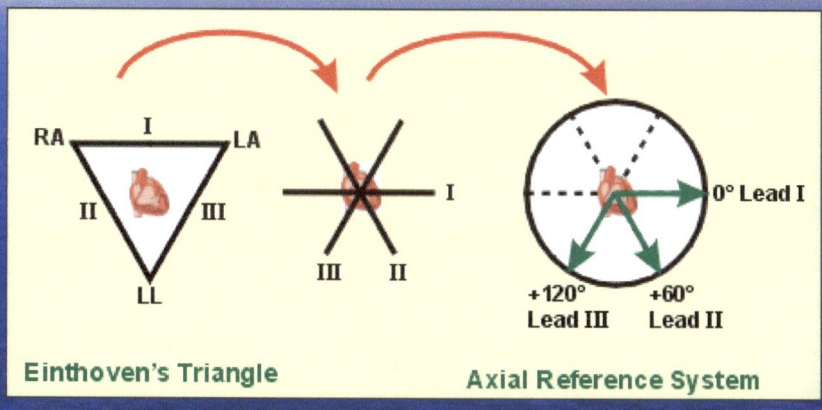

Einthoven's Triangle   Axial Reference System

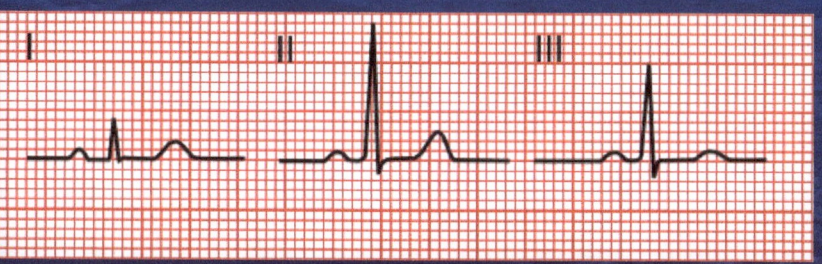

The Augmented Leads Add Much.

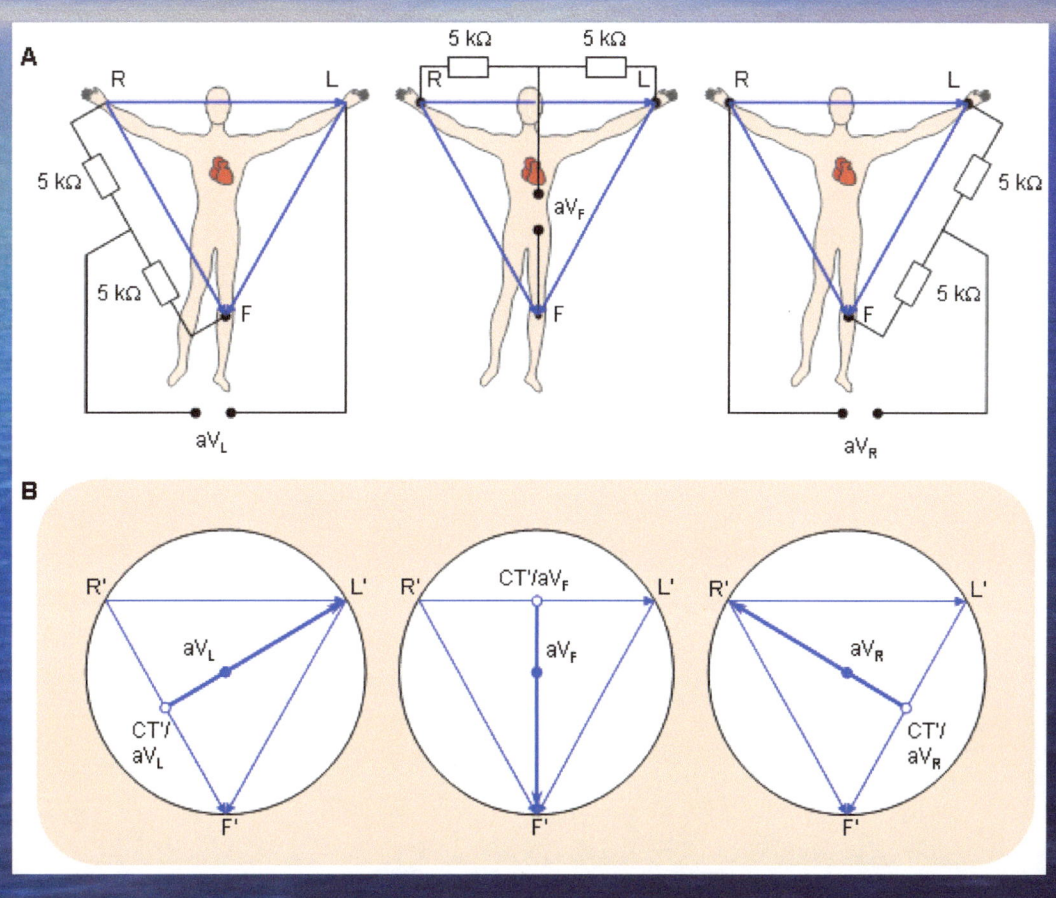

Augmented Limb Leads

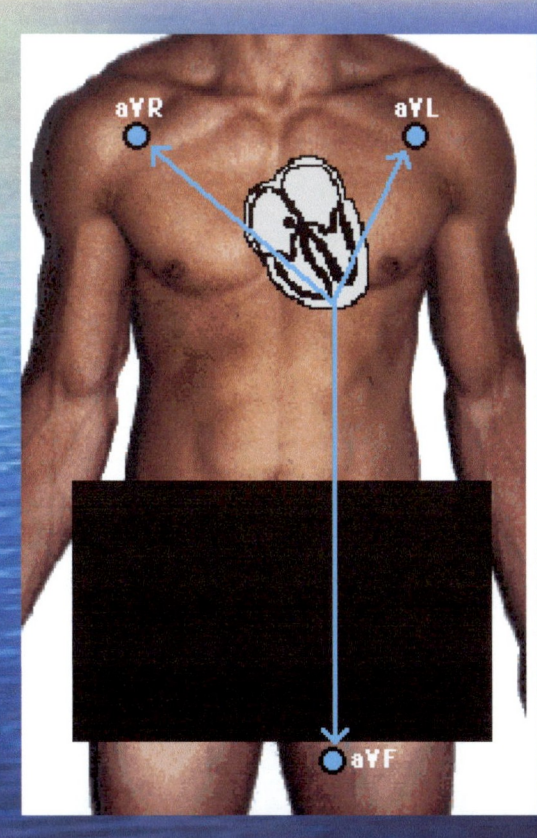
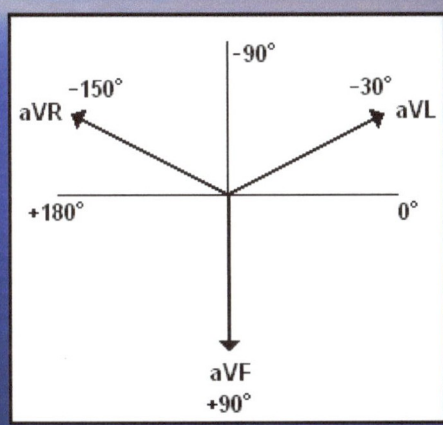
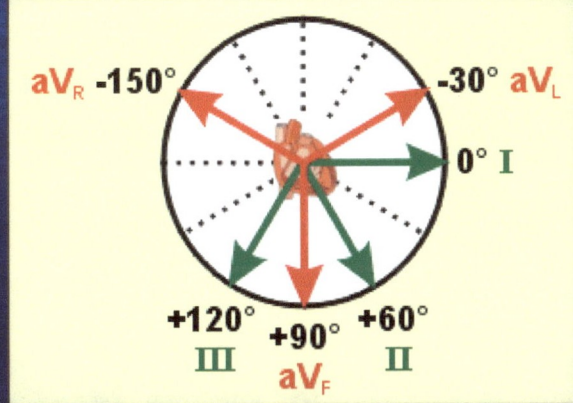

The addition of the augmented limb leads adds to our information on axis orientation, information about high lateral (aVL) and inferior (aVF) myocardium.

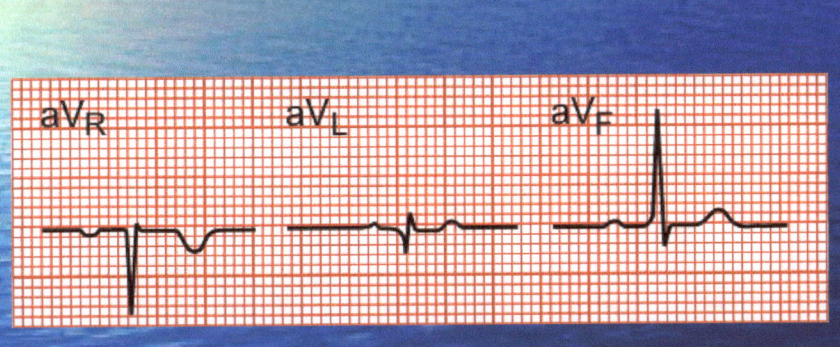
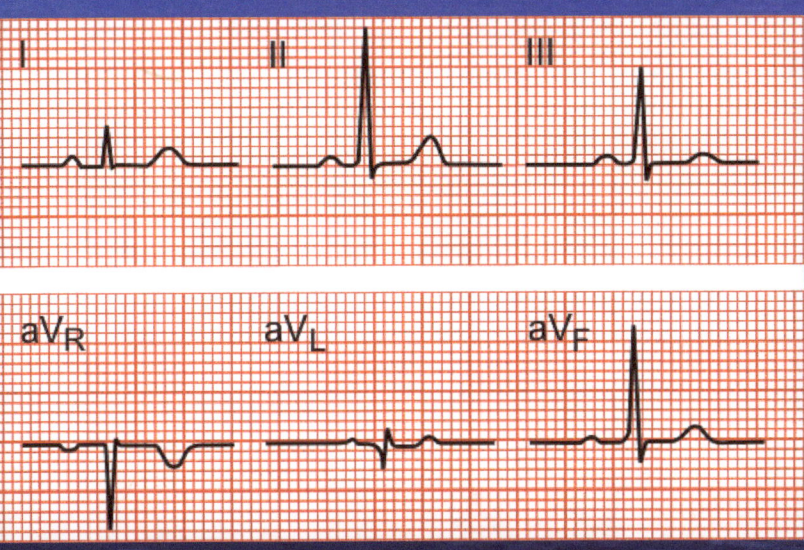

Resting Electrocardiogram.

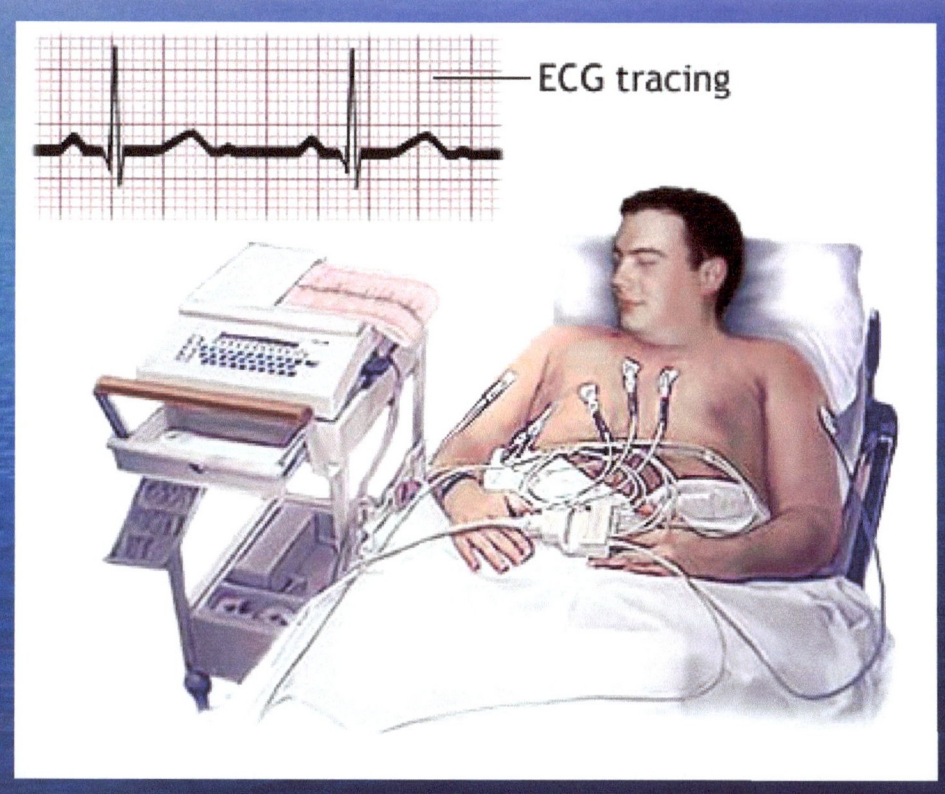

What Does an ECG Actually Represent?

- The electrical activity of the millions of heart cells undergoing depolarization and repolarization resulting from ions moving across the cellular membranes.
- The appearance (deflection) of these moving ions on the electrocardiogram, is dependent upon the positioning of patches on the body allowing us to assign negative and positive leads to measure these changes in membrane polarity.

Timing of the Electrical Activity of the Heart.

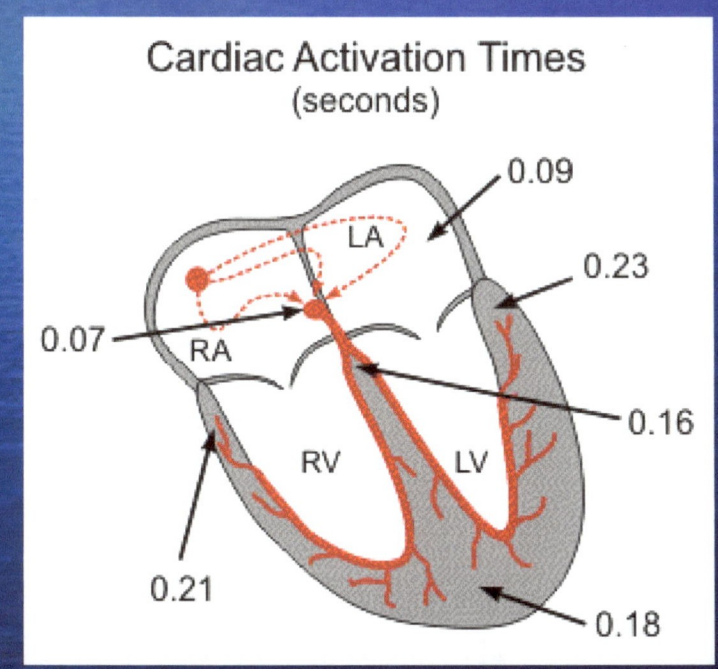

A Standard Electrocardiogram is used to tell us where you're going & which direction you're heading.

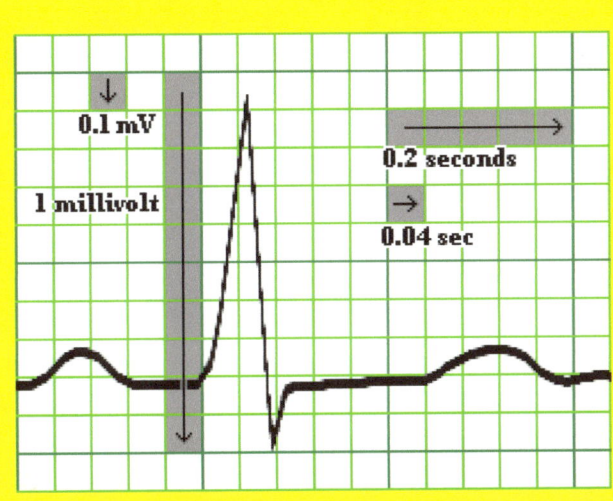
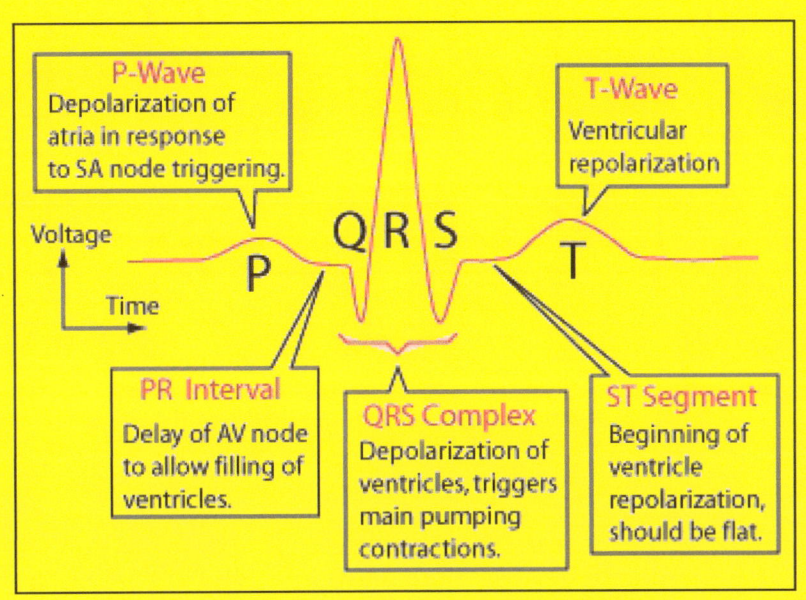

What are the Intervals & Segments?

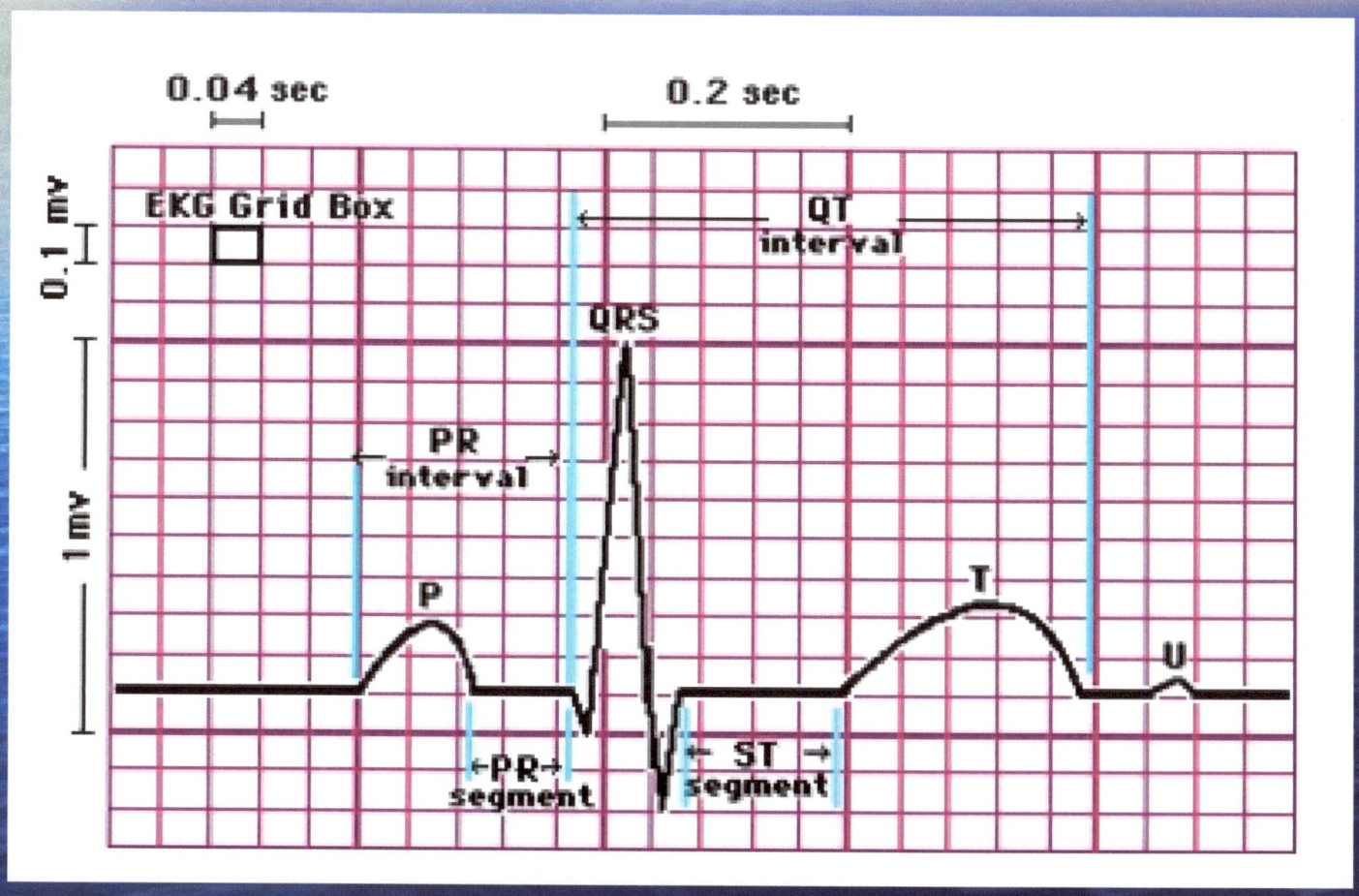

Does Anyone Know Why the Waves have the Names they do?

Bonus Question:
What were the original names for PQRST?

Different leads with have different perspectives.

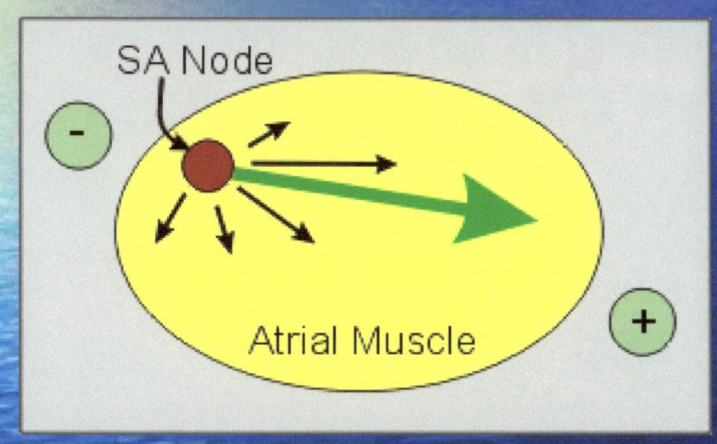
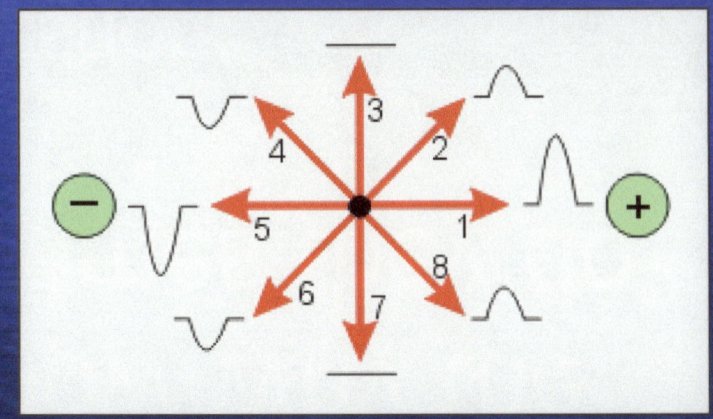

Lead II shows upright P-waves if the P-wave is initiated at the SA node.

The same lead will show different patterns depending upon the origin of the impulse.

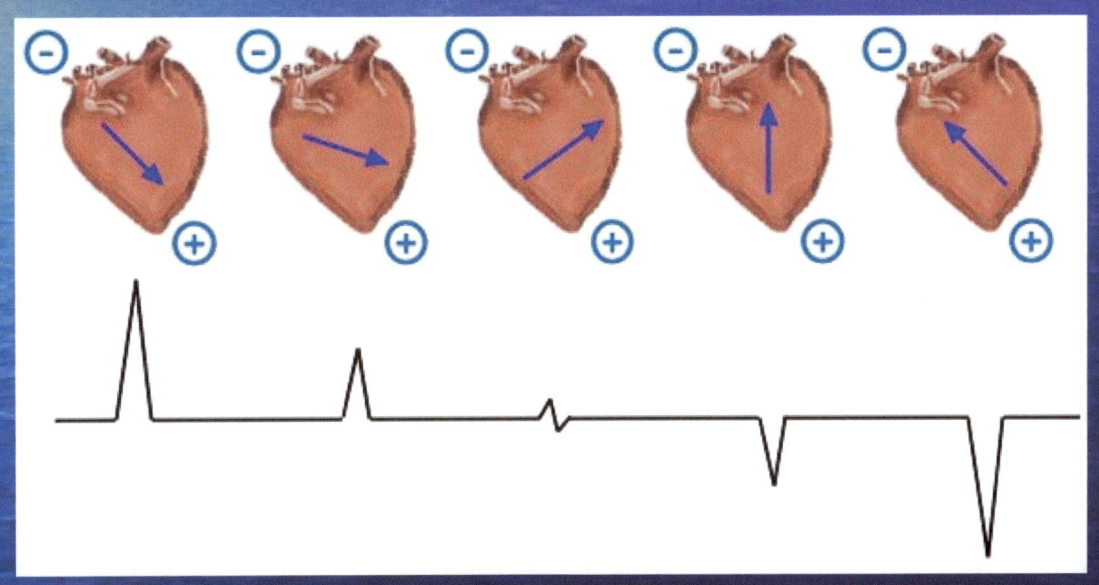

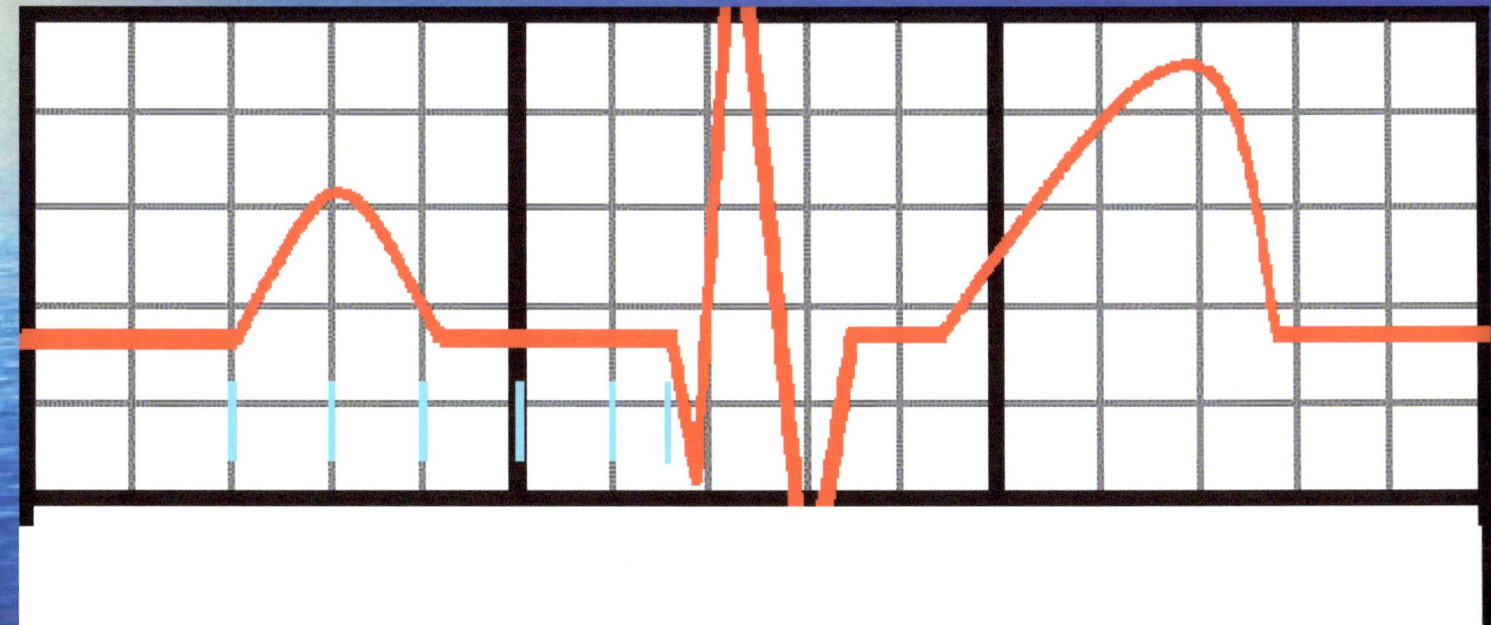

All Standardized Values are Based Upon the Limb Leads.

- PR interval
  - Normal is 0.12 to 0.20 seconds
    - (120-200 mSec)
  - Abnormal
    - Short PR (< 120 mSec)
      - Pre-excitation syndrome
      - AV Junctional Rhythm (retrograde p-waves)
      - Ectopic Atrial Rhythms (waveform dependent upon origin)
      - Normal Variant

What's the PR Interval & Rhythm?

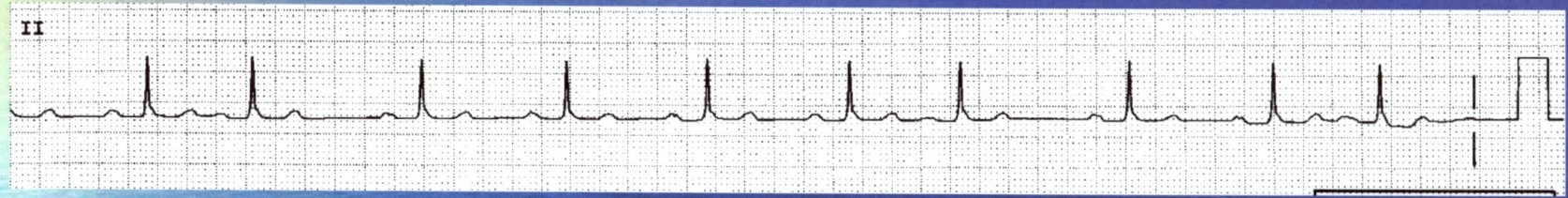

- Is it Sinus?
- Is the Rhythm regular?
  - What is the Rhythm?
- What is the PR Interval?

What is the PR interval?
What is the Rhythm?

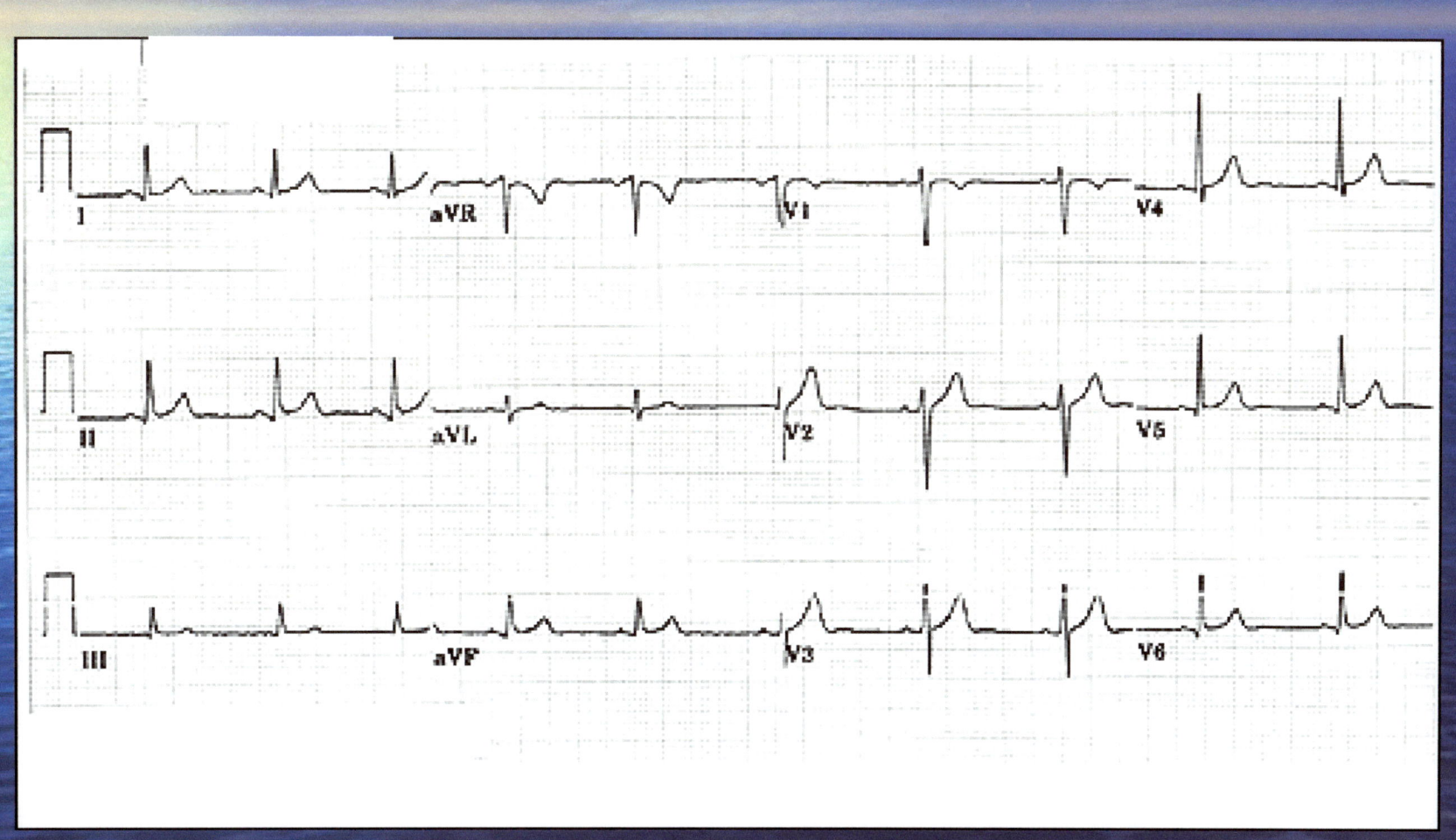

What is the PR Interval and Rhythm?

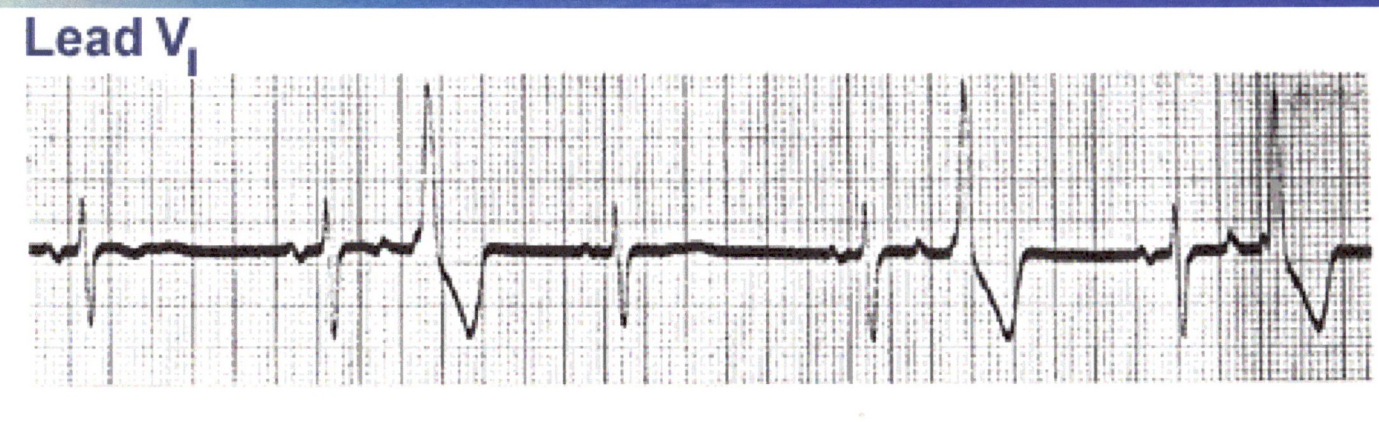

What is the PR Interval and the Rhythm?

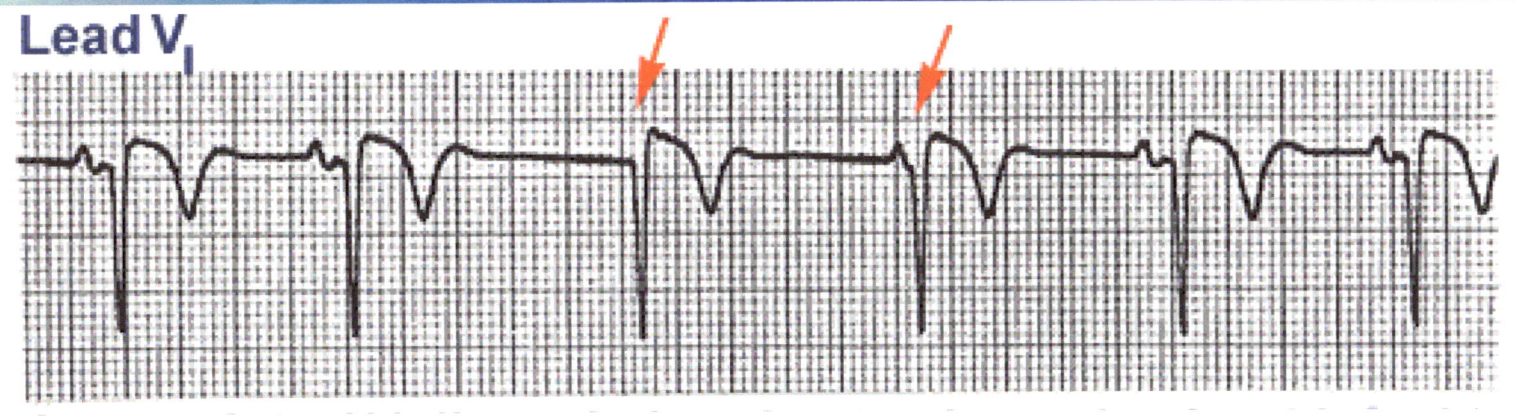

Any Guesses?

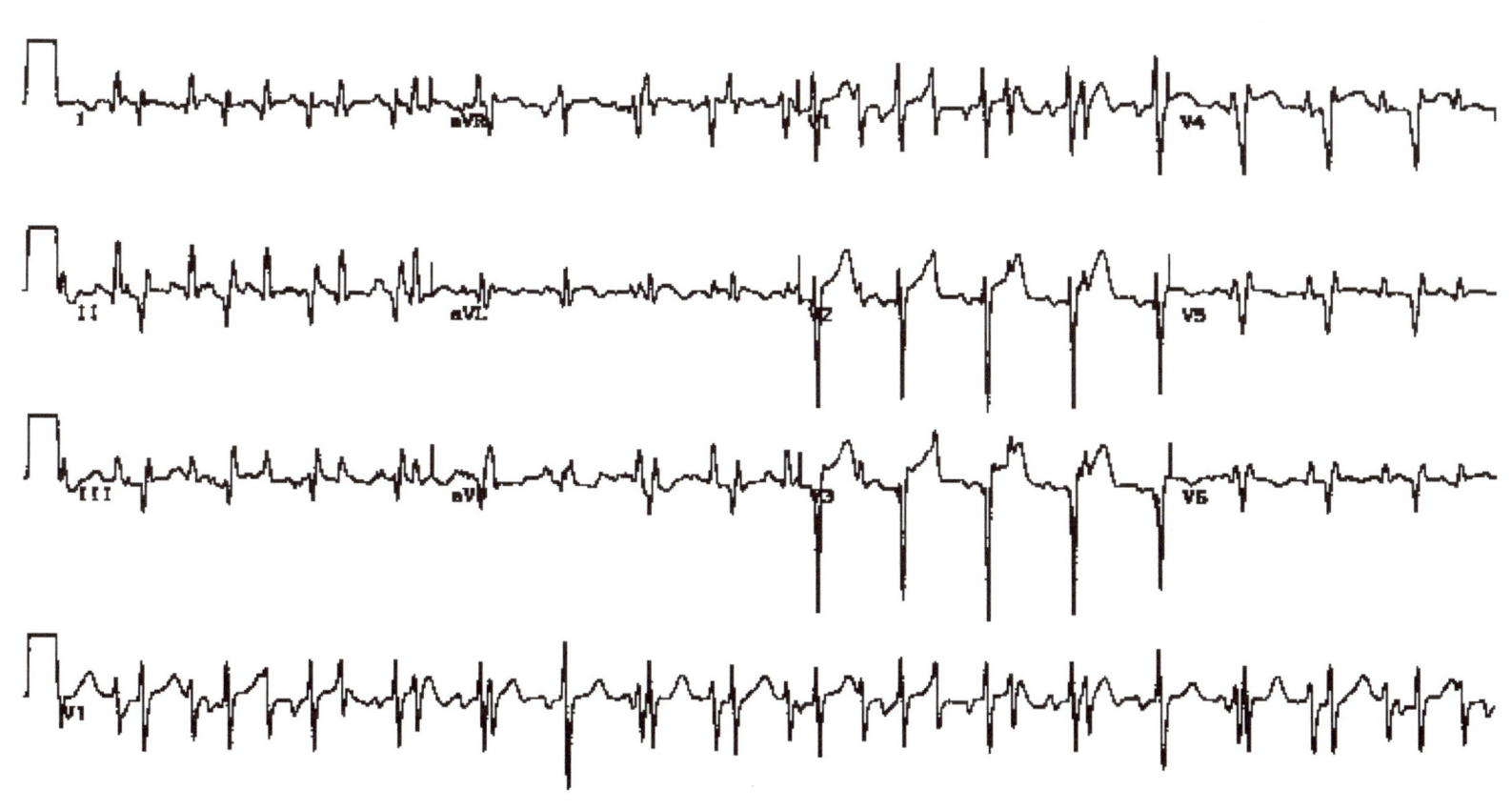

PR Interval (cont):

- PR interval
  - Abnormal
    - Long PR (> 200 mSec)
      - 1° AV Block (PR usually constant)
      - Intra-atrial conduction delay (uncommon)
      - Slowed AV conduction (most common)
      - Slowed His conduction (rare)
      - Slowed conduction in bundle branch when opposite branch is blocked

PR Interval (cont):

- PR interval
  - Abnormal
    - 2° AV Block (PR may be normal or prolonged)
      - Type I (Wenckebach)
        - PR gets progressively longer and RR progressively shorter until the p-wave is finally dropped.
      - Type II (Mobitz)
        - Fixed PR interval where p-wave is suddenly dropped.
    - 3° AV Block
      - Also known as AV dissociation
      - Atrial rate (P-P) constant & Ventricular rate (R-R) constant
        - But the rates are different.

First Degree Atrioventricular Block

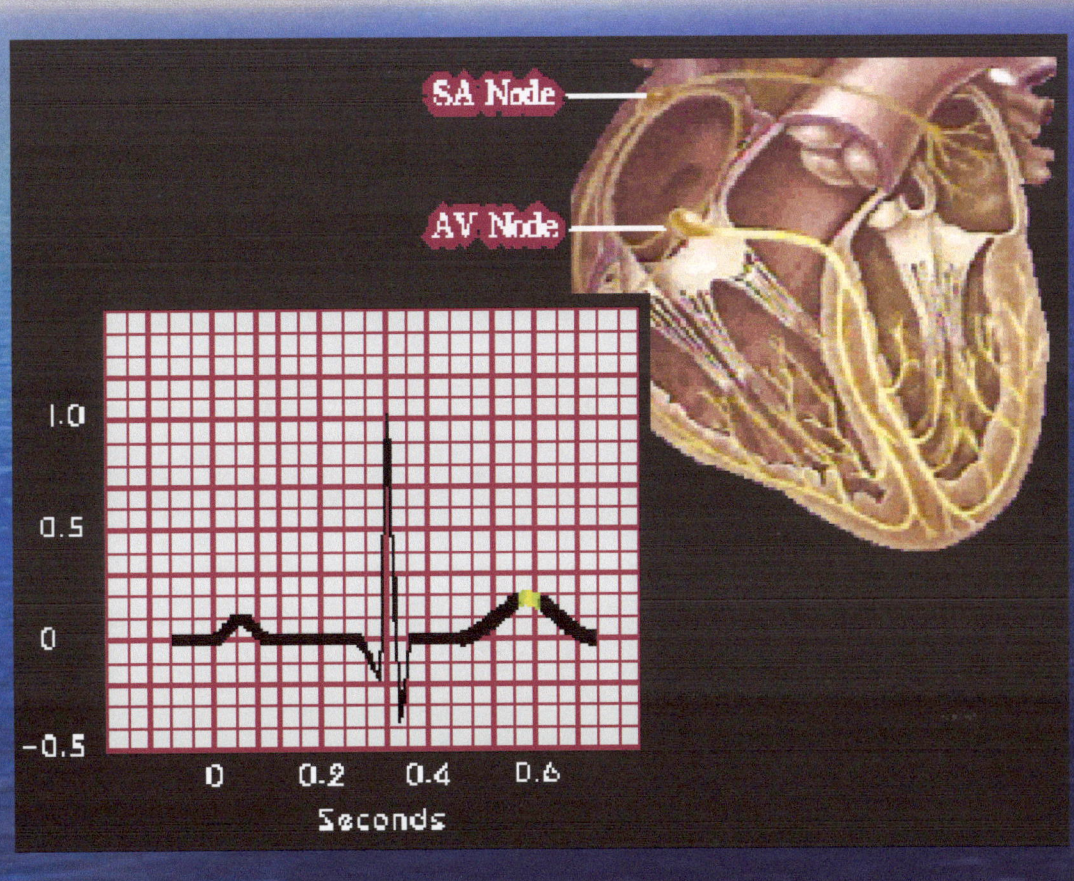

What is the PR Interval and What is the Rhythm?

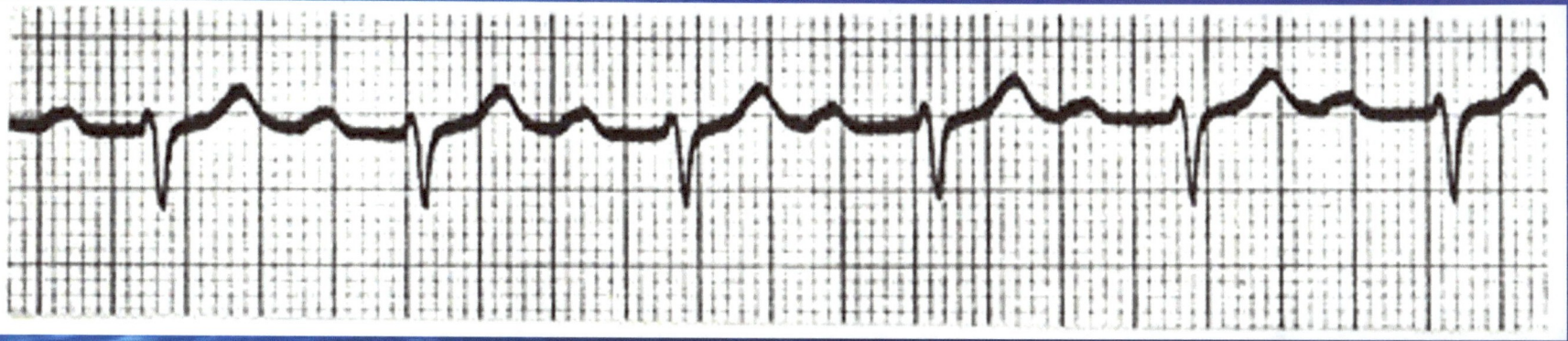

What is the PR Interval and What is the Rhythm?

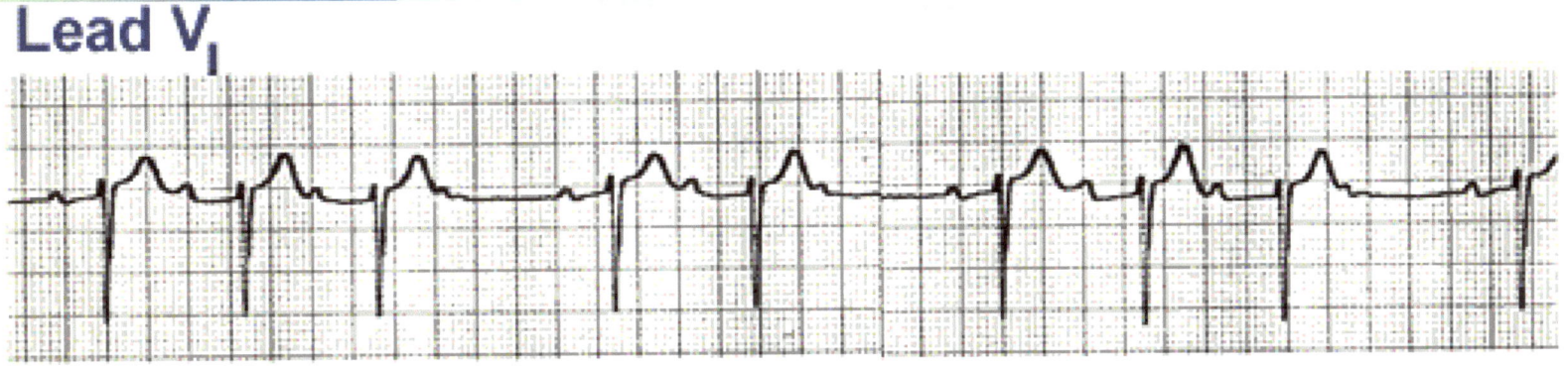

Lecture 2:
What Have we Learned to date?

- Basic principles of cells and capacitors.
- What determines a positive and negative deflection in a lead.
- What the limb and precordial leads represent.
- How to measure PR intervals.
- Now we will move onto QRS.
  – Axis & Duration.

Action Potential of Bundle of His & Myocardium.

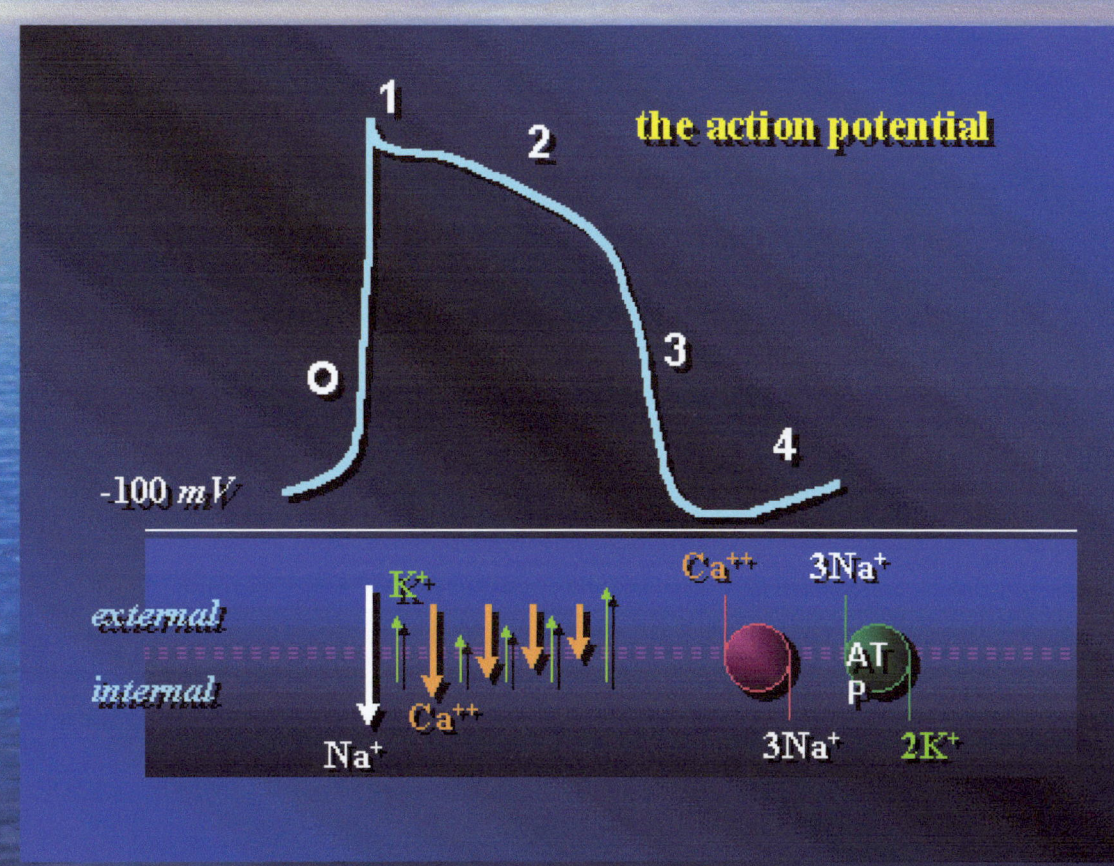

The His-Purkinje system: Slowing of fascicles or bundles causes a shift in the QRS axis.

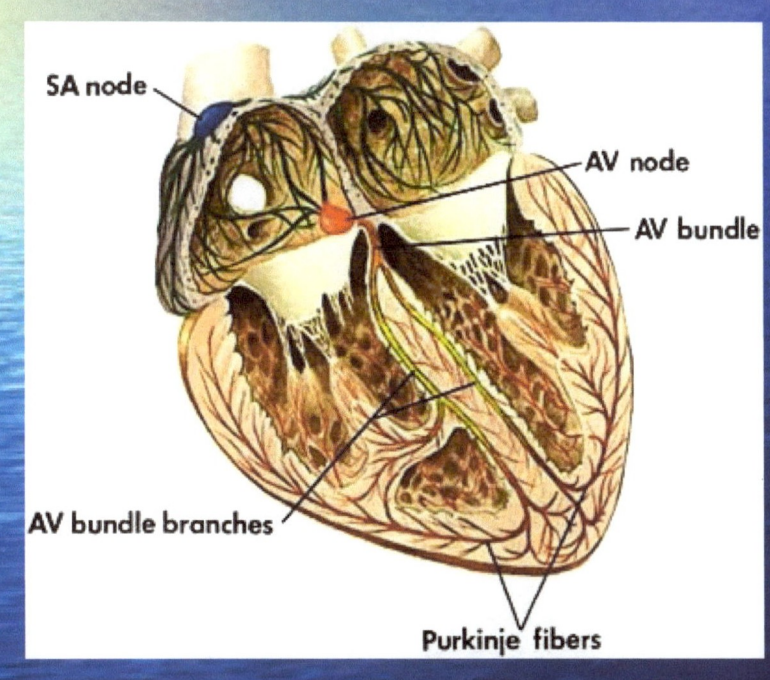
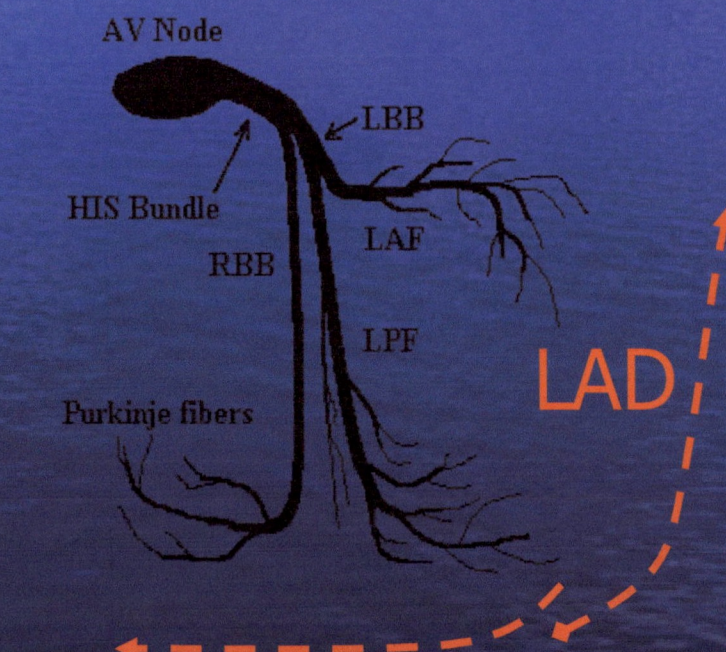

The Normal QRS Axis.

- By near-consensus, the normal QRS axis is defined as ranging from -30° to +90°.

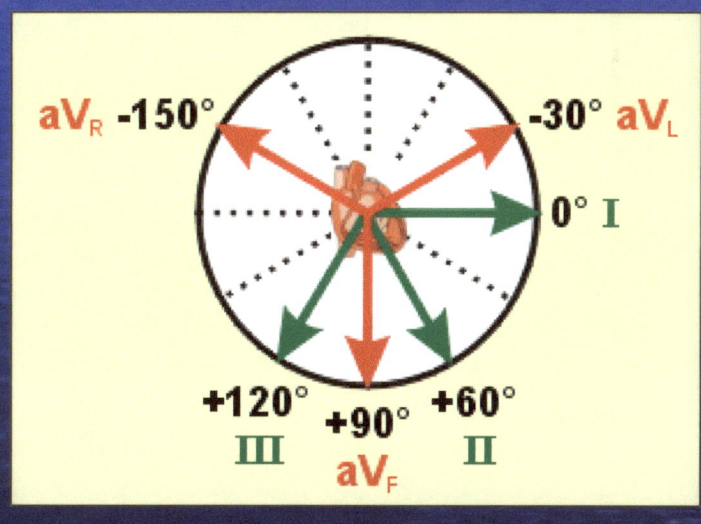

The QRS Axis

- −30° to −90° is referred to as a left axis deviation (LAD)

- +90° to +180° is referred to as a right axis deviation (RAD)

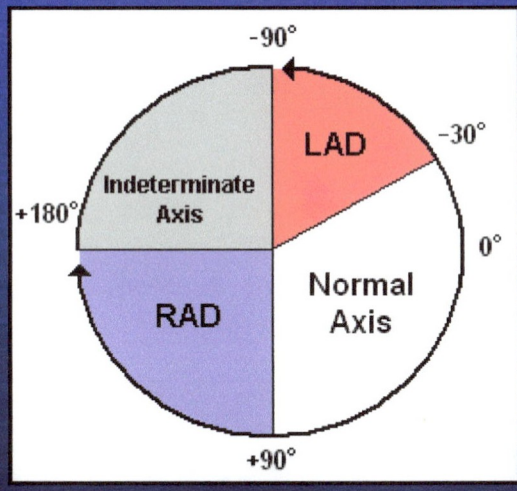

The QRS Axis – Tells us what and where something is happening in the His-Purkinje System.

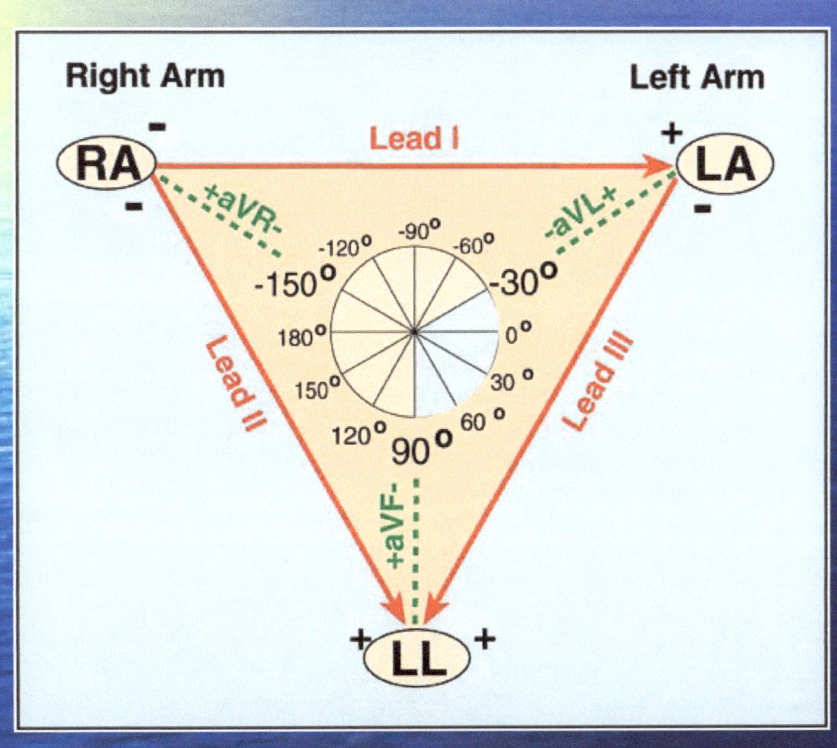

- Lead I (180° to 0°)
- Lead aVR (-150° to 30°)
- Lead II (-120° to 60°)
- Lead aVF (-90° to 90°)
- Lead III (-60° to 120°)
- Lead aVL (150° to -30°)

The His-Purkinje system: Slowing of fascicles or bundles causes a shift in the QRS axis.

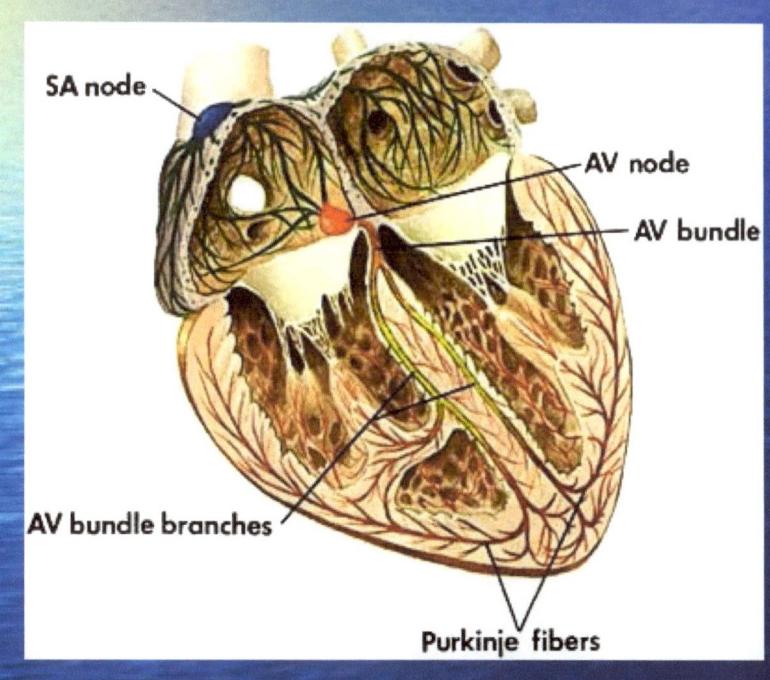
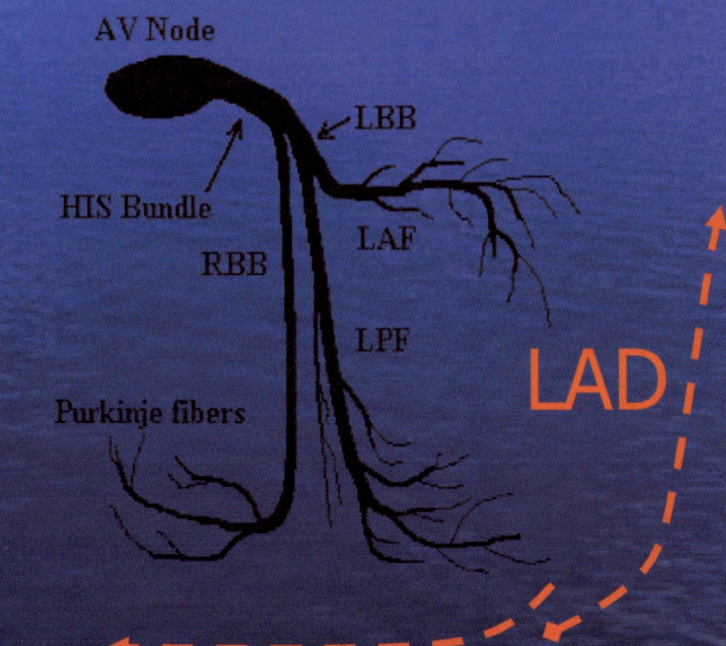

The Isoelectric approach to QRS Orientation. You can't tell if it's normal if you don't know how to figure it out!

- 1. Find the lead which is isoelectric
  - The above and below baseline are equal.
  - If there is no isoelectric lead (up in every lead), the QRS is indeterminate (normal variant).
- 2. The QRS is perpendicular to this lead.
  - If no single lead fits this, there will be two that are nearly isoelectric (30° apart), the perpendicular is midway between them.
- 3. Now you need to decide which perpendicular direction is correct by using the other leads.

Normal (0°): QRS Axis

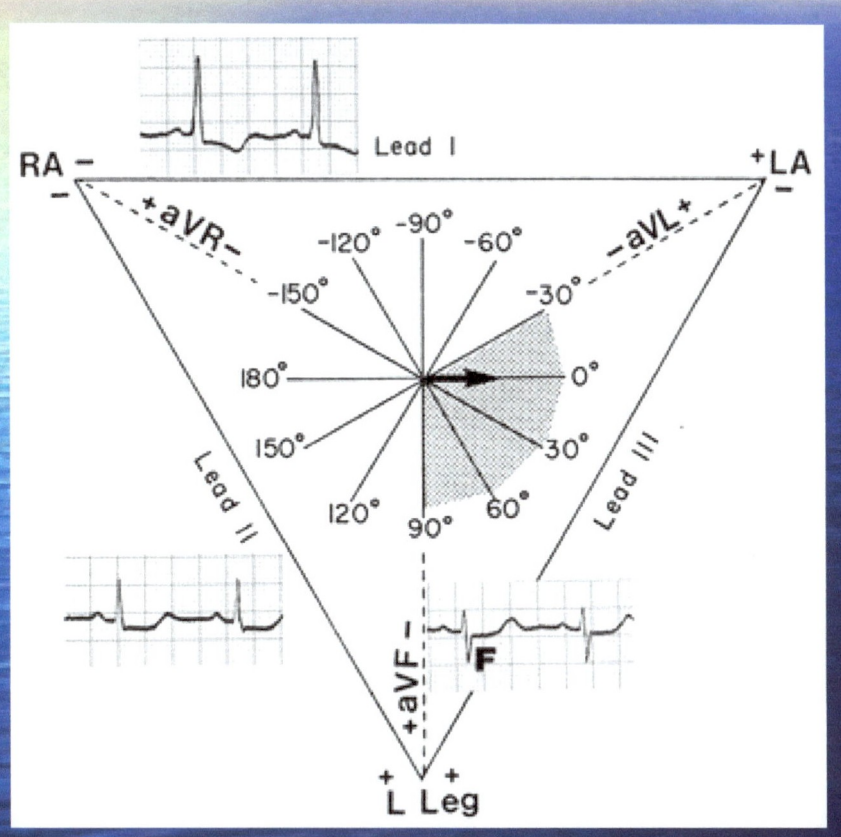

- aVF is isoelectric
  - So QRS axis is 90° from this.
  - Either 0° or 180°
- QRS is positive in I
- QRS is positive in II
- Therefore
  - QRS axis = 0°
- Normal Axis

LAD (-60°): aVR is isoelectric.

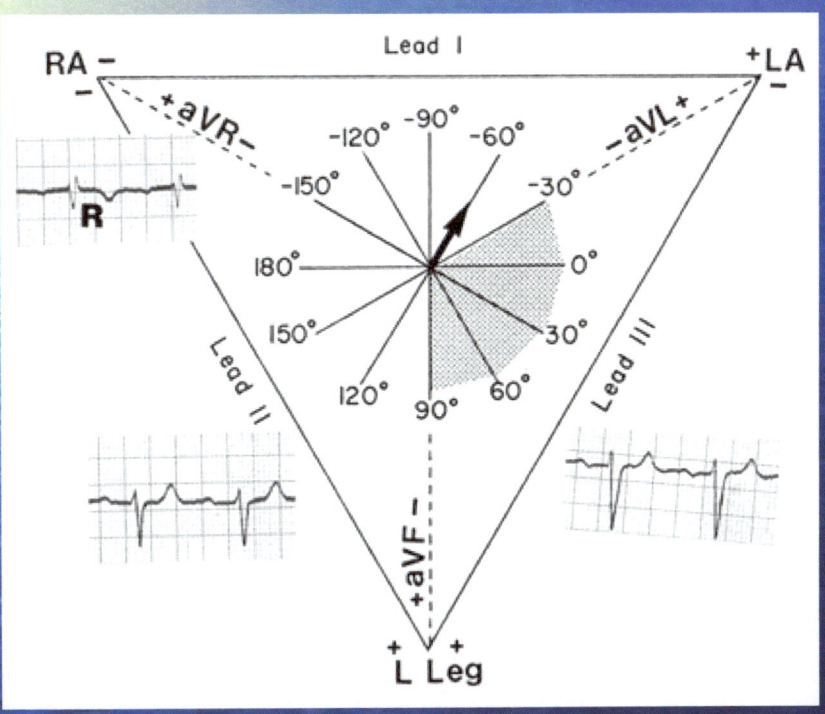

- aVR is isoelectric
  - So QRS axis is 90° from this.
  - Either -60° or 120°
- QRS is negative in III
- QRS is negative in II
- Therefore
  - QRS axis = -60°
- LAD

RAD (+120°): aVR isoelectric.

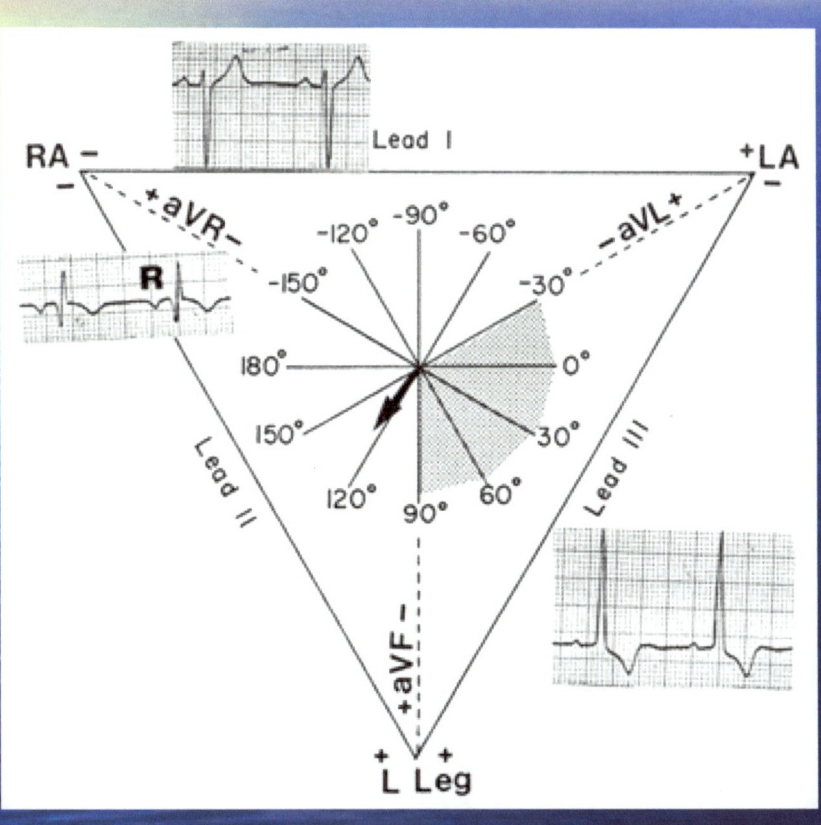

- aVR is ~ isoelectric
  - So QRS axis is 90° from this.
  - Either -60° or 120°
- QRS is positive in III
- QRS is negative in I
- Therefore
  - QRS axis = ~ 120°
- RAD

The Quadrant Approach to QRS Orientation.

1. Examine the QRS complex in leads I and aVF to determine if they are predominantly positive or predominantly negative. The combination should place the axis into one of the 4 quadrants below.

2. 2. In the event that LAD is present, examine lead II to determine if this deviation is pathologic. If the QRS in II is predominantly positive, the LAD is non-pathologic (in other words, the axis is normal). If it is predominantly negative, it is pathologic.

		Lead aVF	
		Positive	Negative
Lead I	Positive	Normal Axis	LAD
	Negative	RAD	Indeterminate Axis

What is the QRS axis?

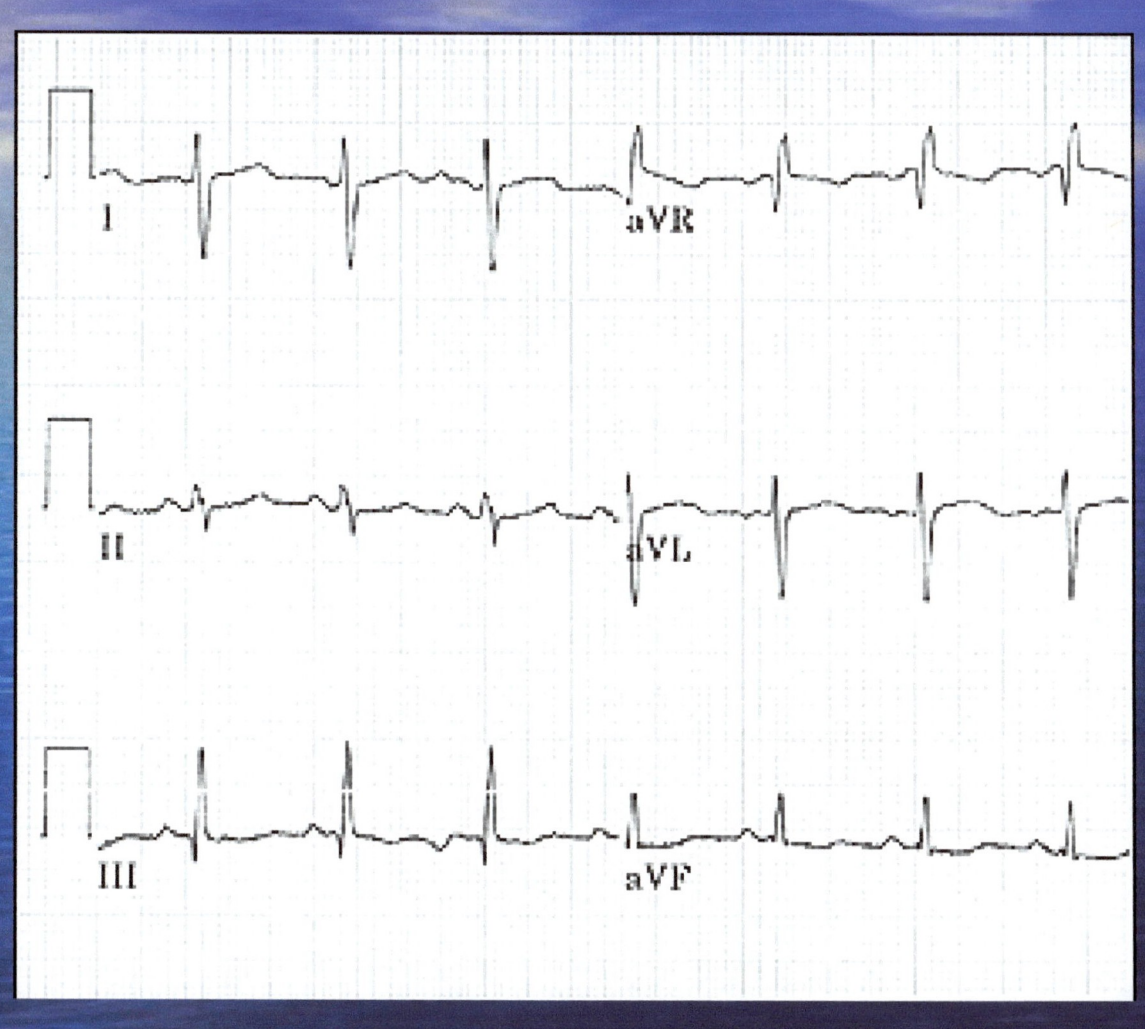

What is this QRS axis?

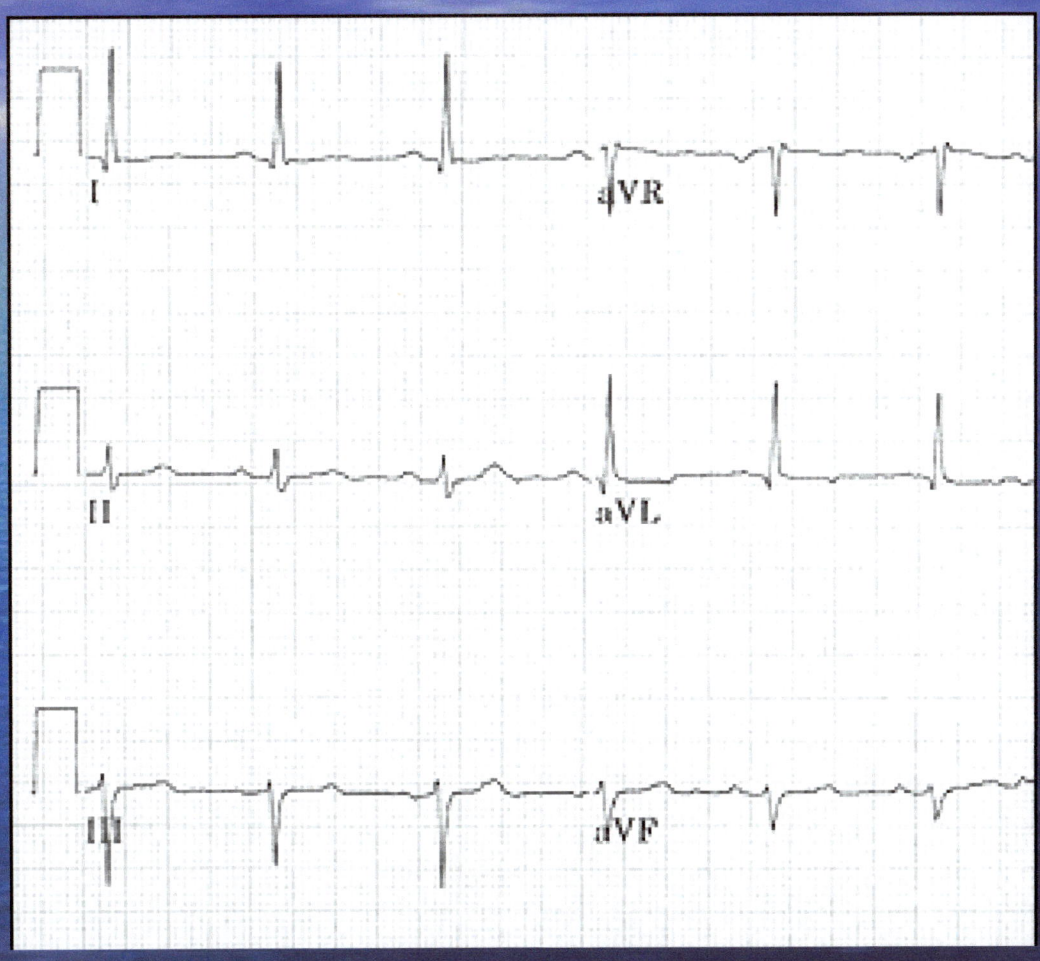

What is this QRS axis?

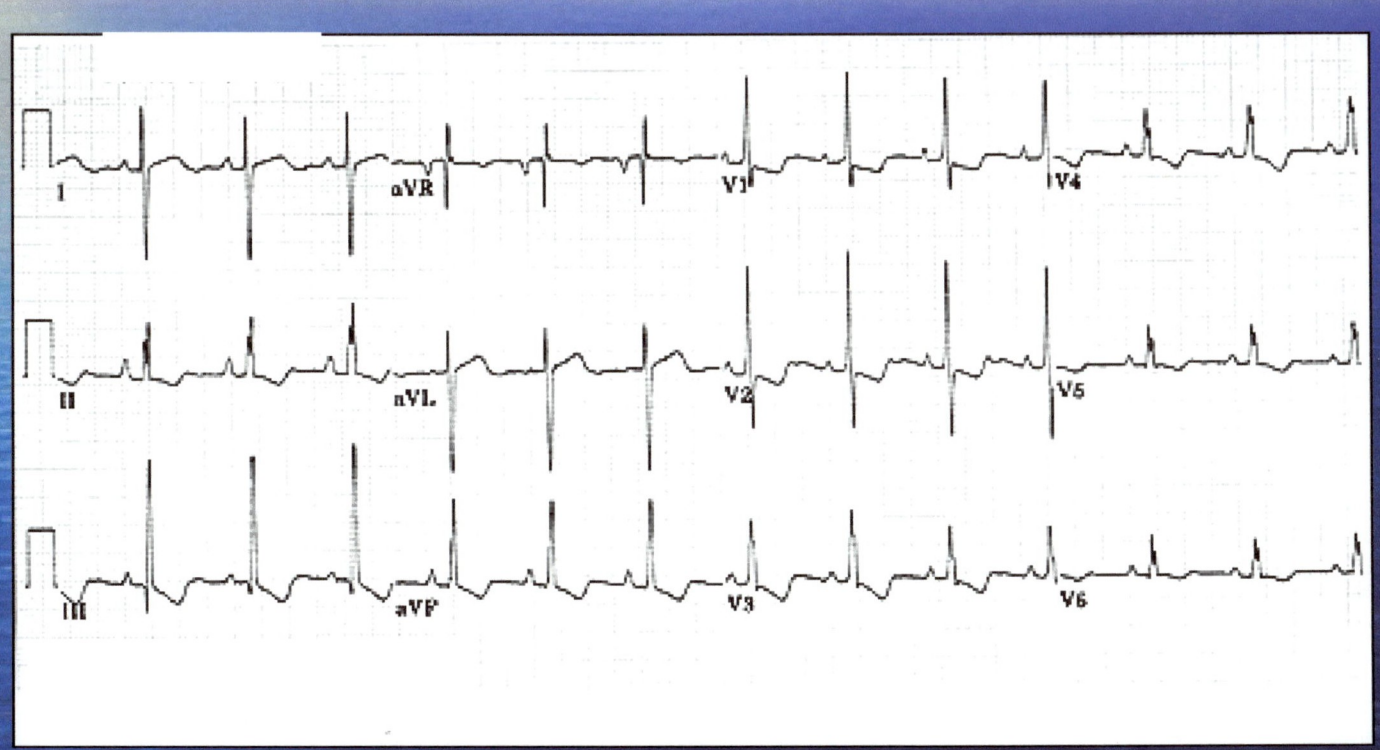

Measuring QRS Duration: The length of ventricular depolarization.

- Normal
  - 0.06 to 0.120 sec (60 to 120 mSec)
    - True normal is 60 to 100 mSec
    - Intraventricular conduction delay (IVCD) is 100 to 120 mSec.
      - Sometimes broken down as incomplete rBBB or incomplete LBBB.
      - Fascicular blocks
        - Left anterior (LAD, qI, sIII) fascicular block
        - Left posterior (rBBB, sI, qIII) fascicular block

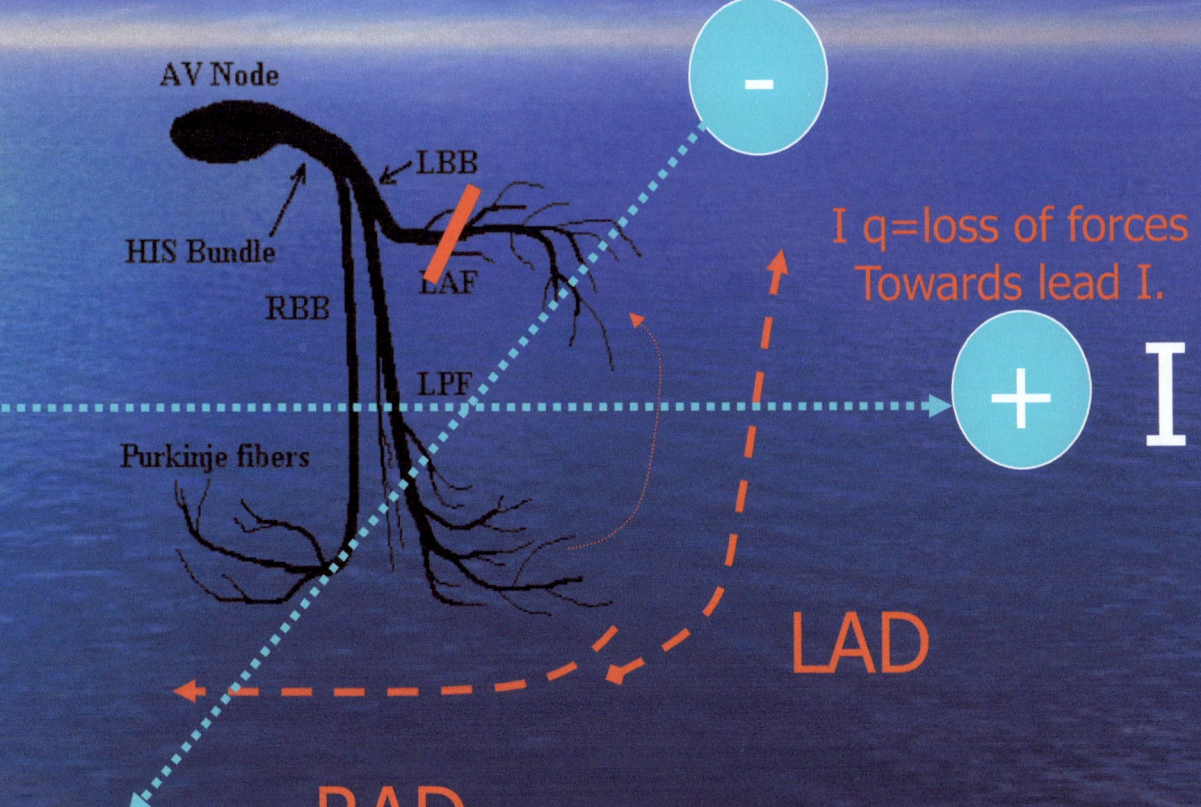

Left Anterior Fascicular Block

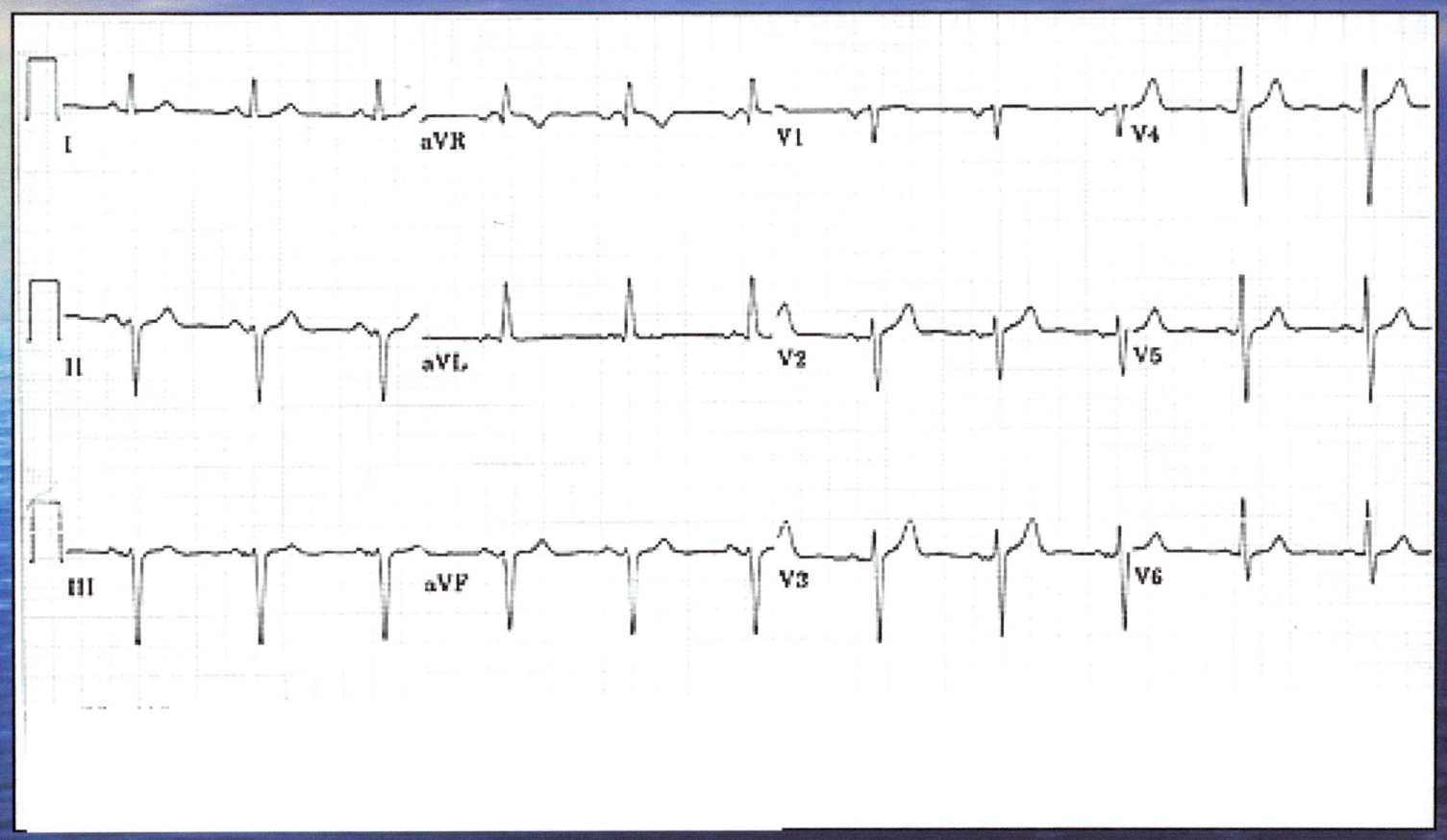

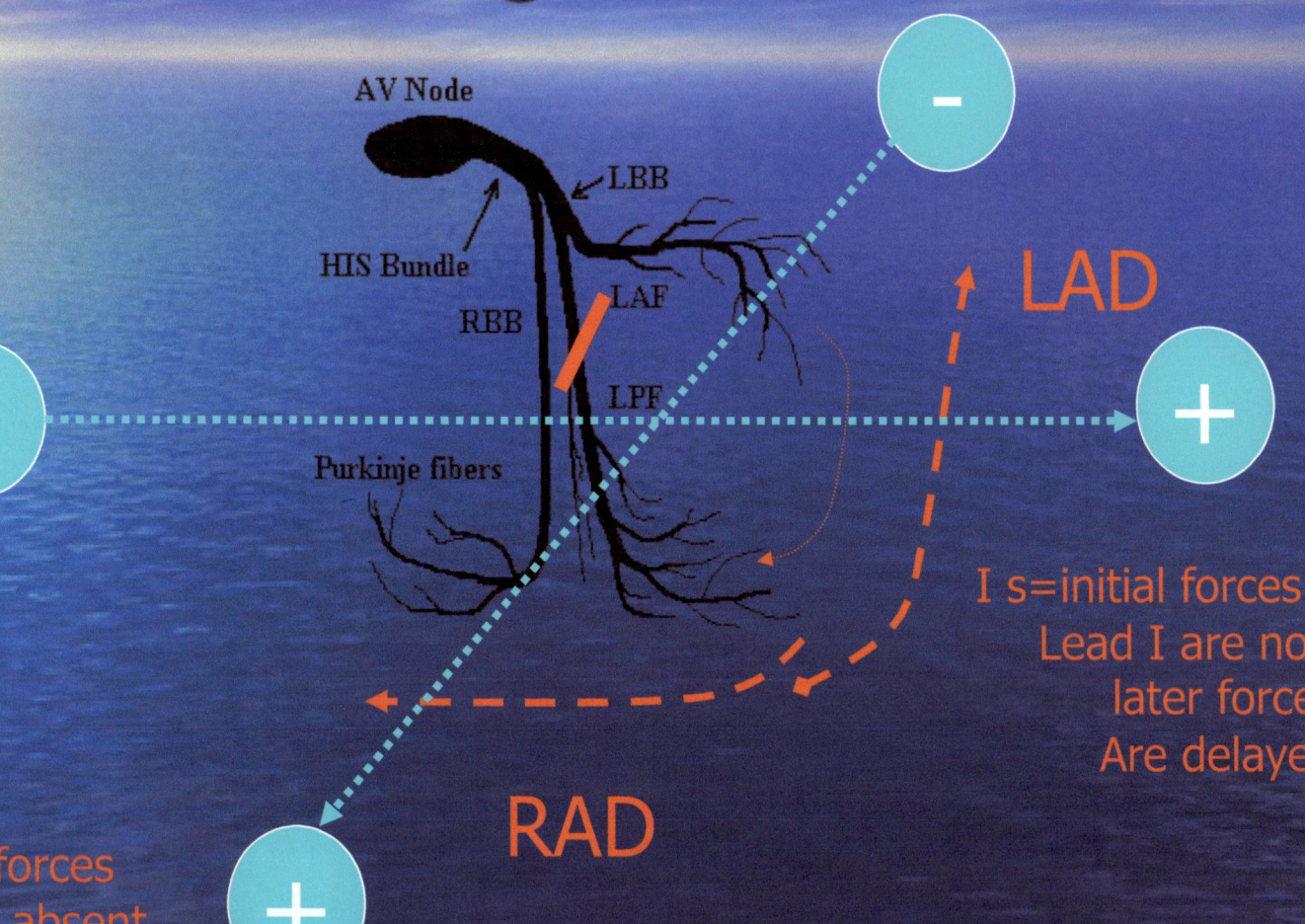

Left Posterior Fascicular Block

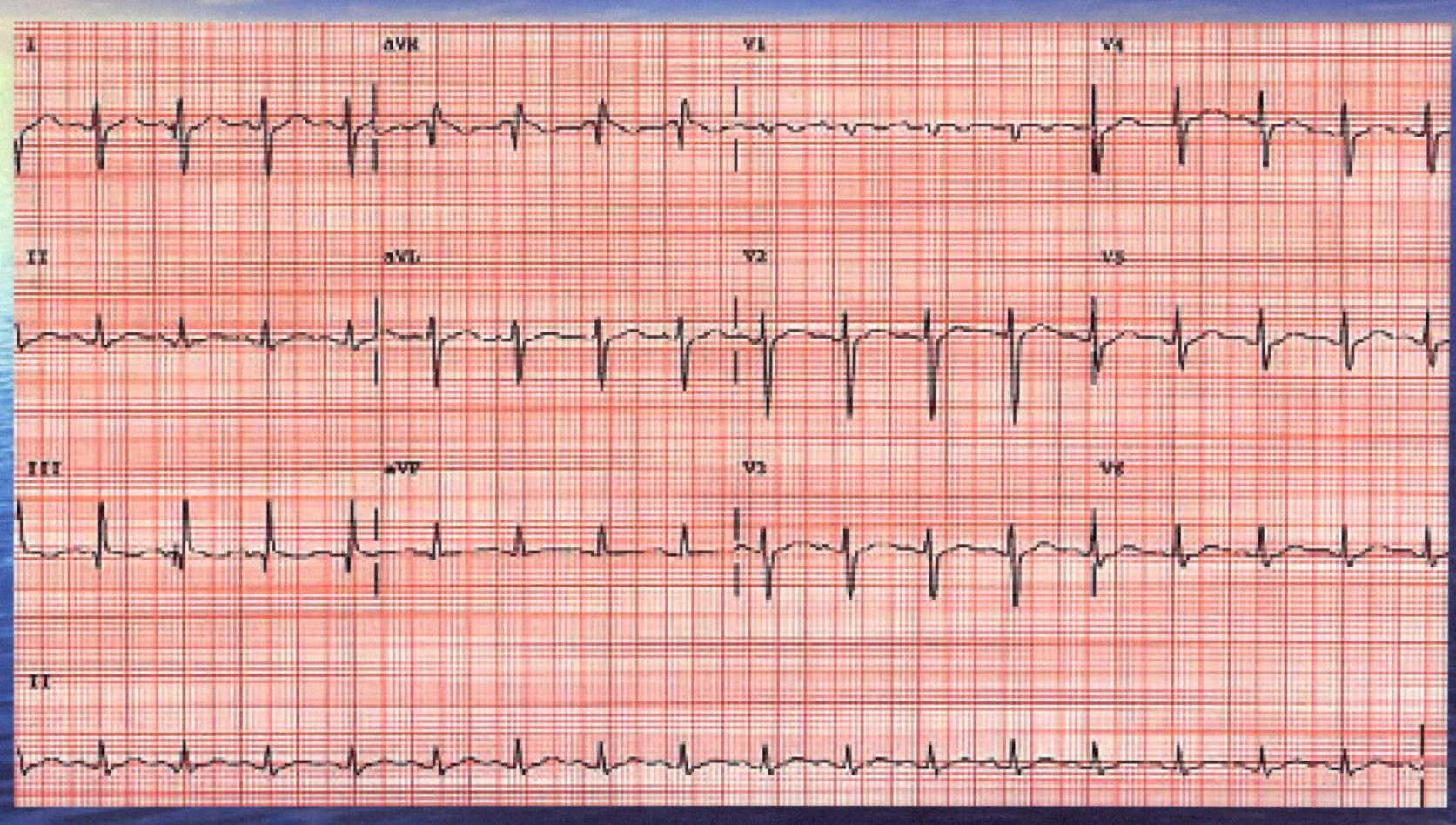

Measuring QRS Duration (cont):

- Prolonged QRS > 120 mSec
  - rBBB
  - LBBB
    - Not an IVCD (up to 120 mSec)
  - Ectopic ventricular rhythms
    - VPBs
    - Ventricular Pacemaker
      - (pacing, sensing, response)
- Unique waves
  - Delta, Osborne, Epsilon, Brugada

Bundle-Branch Injury

- The His-Purkinje System.
    - rBBB
        - PACs with aberrancy
        - The right bundle has a longer refractory period than the left bundle. Therefore, an early atrial impulse runs the risk of running into a right bundle which is still refractory thereby slowing the impulse (rBBB) through it.
            - These are therefore rate dependent and show up with increased HR or PACs.
    - LBBB (composed of two separate fascicles)
        - LAFB
        - LPFB

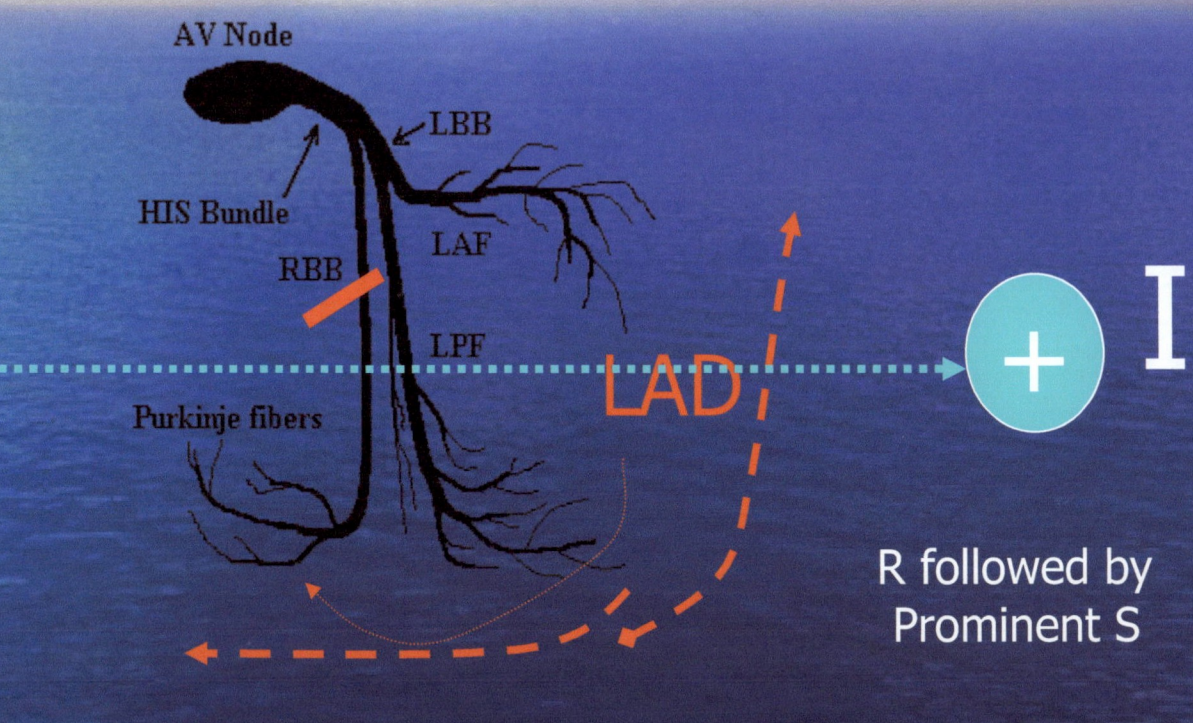

The His-Purkinje system:
The initial force is from left to right across the septum towards V1.

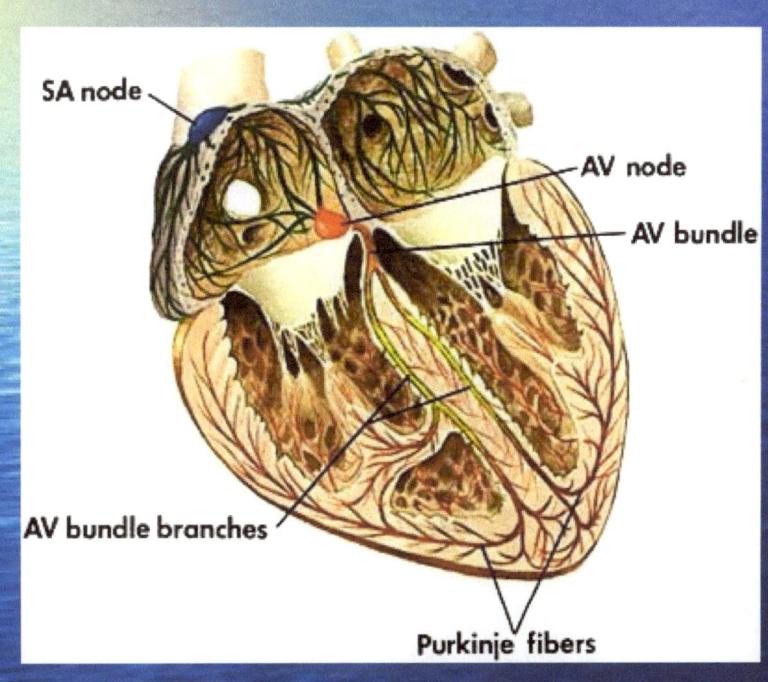

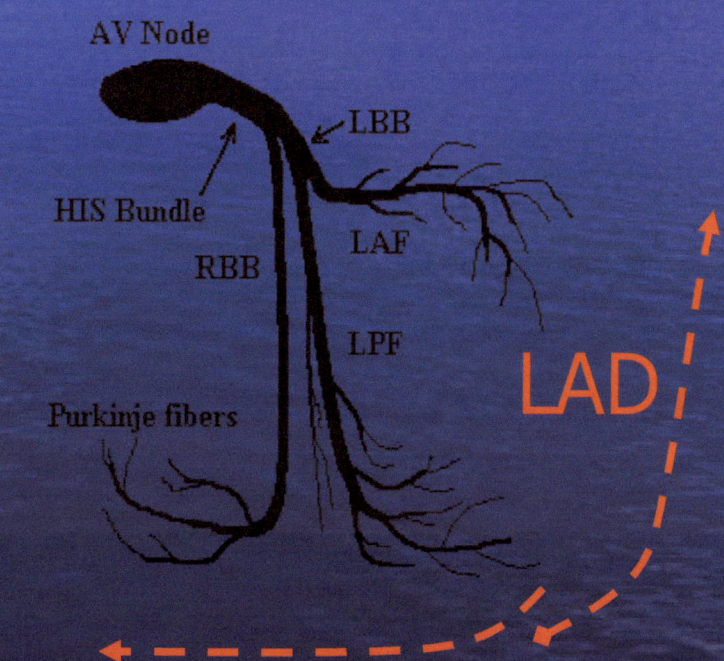

LAD

RAD

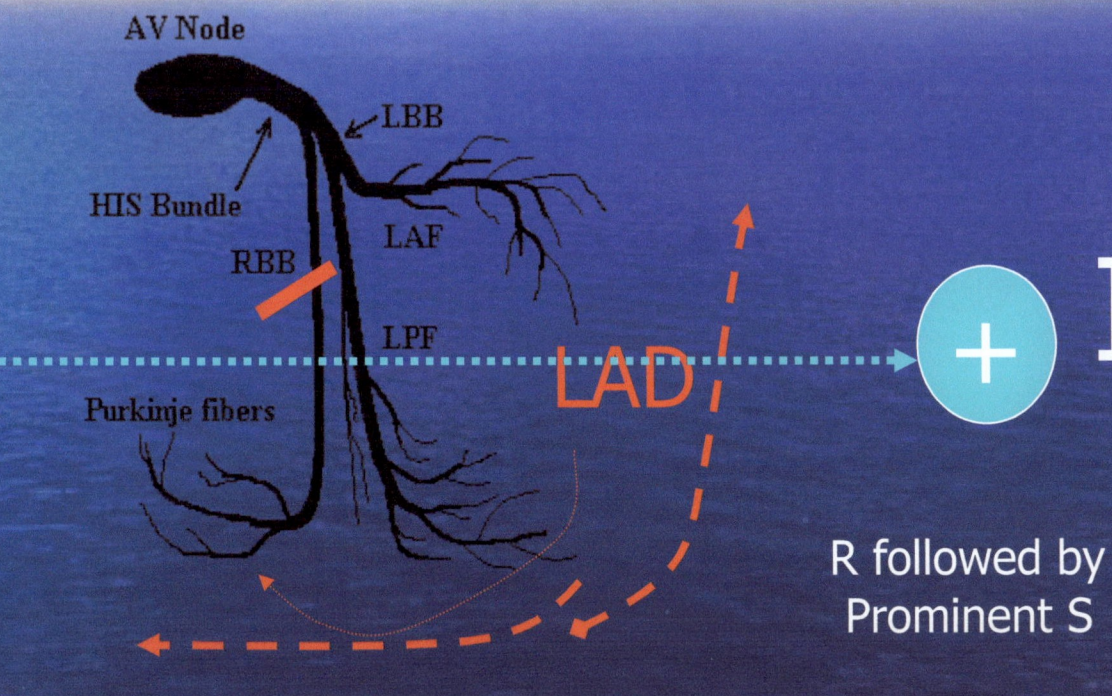

Right Bundle Branch Block

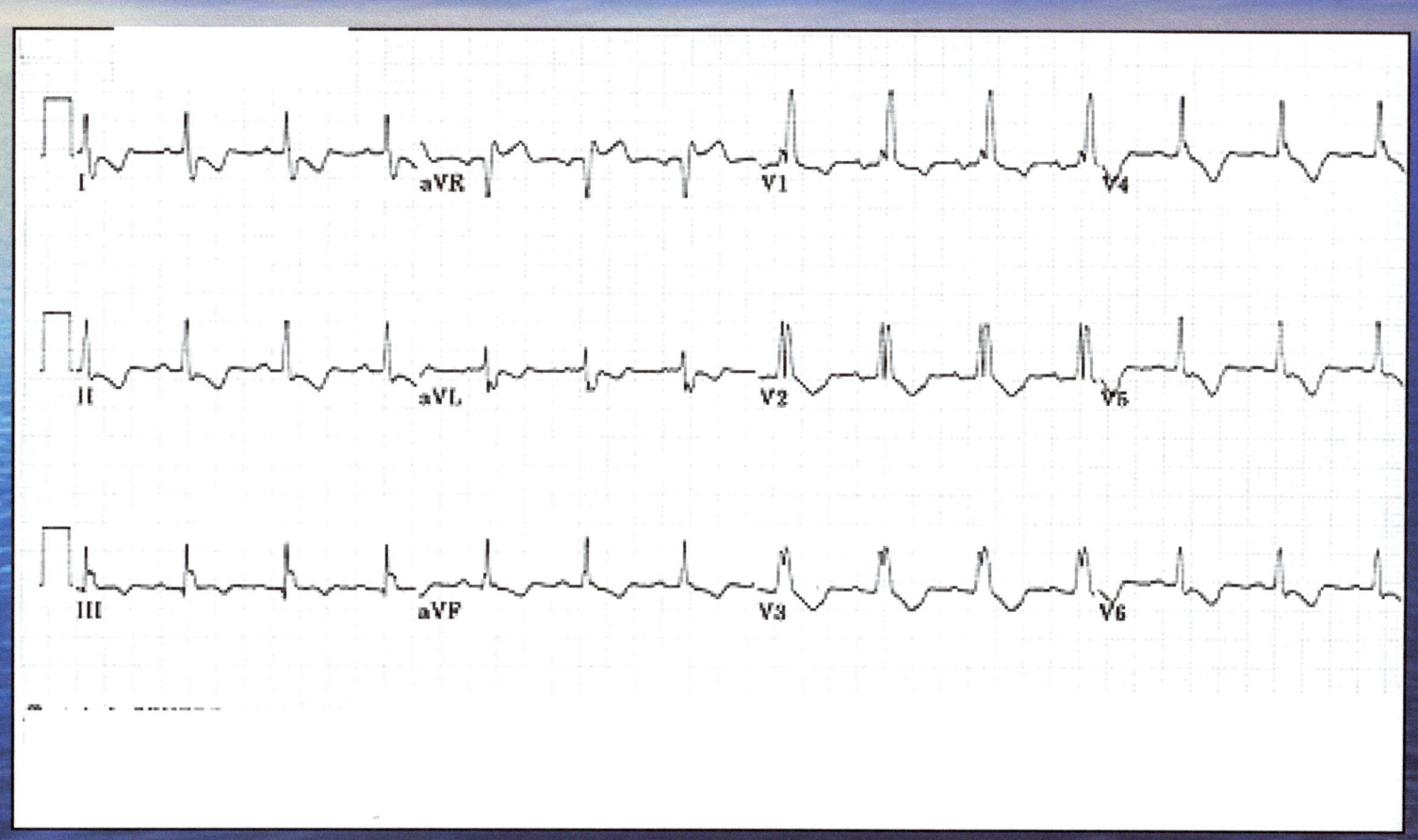

PAC with rBBB

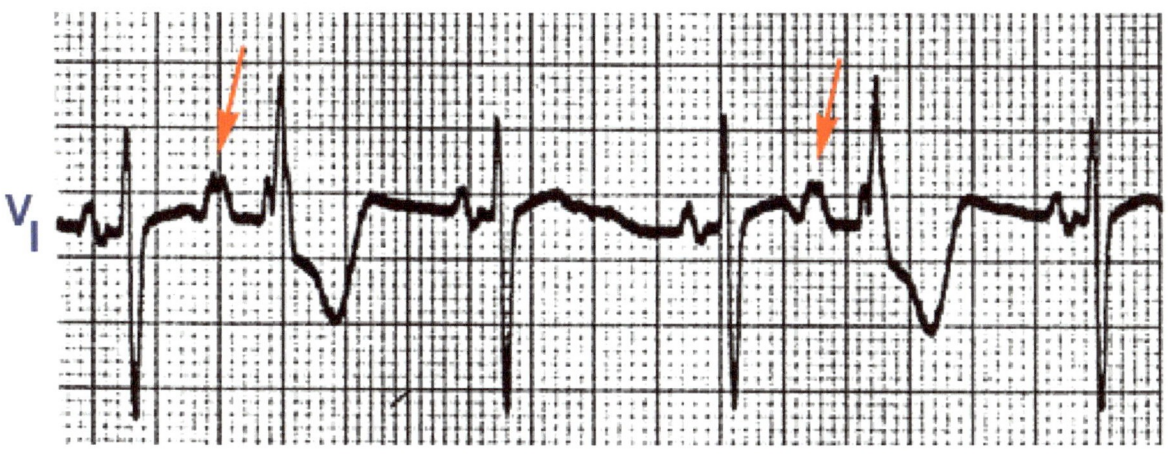

PAC's (arrow) with atypical RBBB aberration

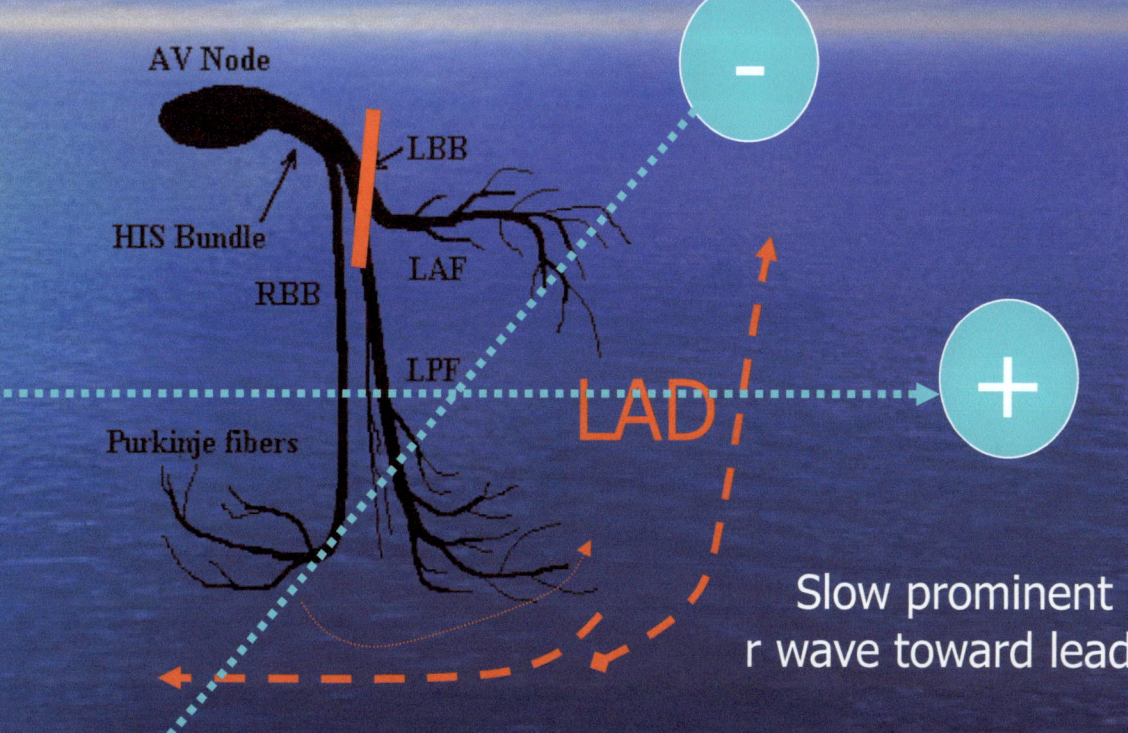

The His-Purkinje system:
The initial force is from left to right across the septum towards V1.

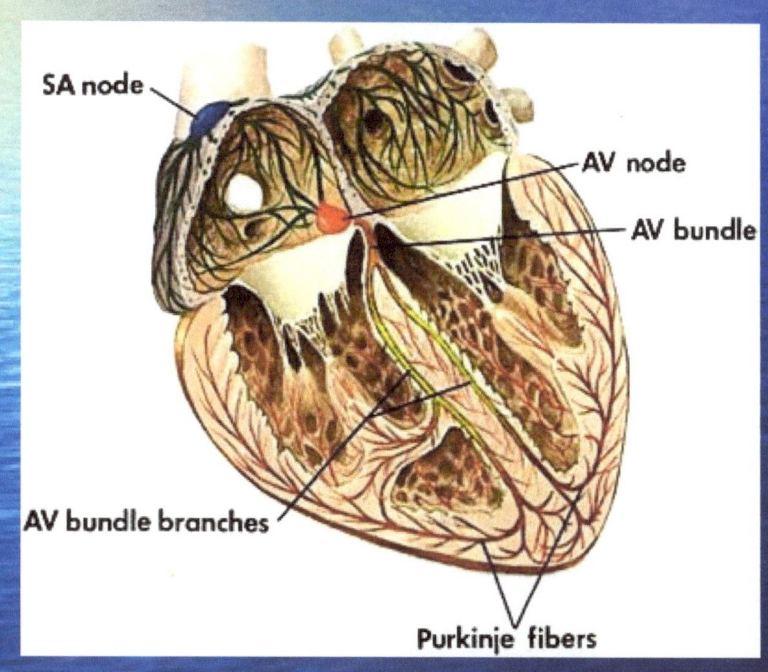

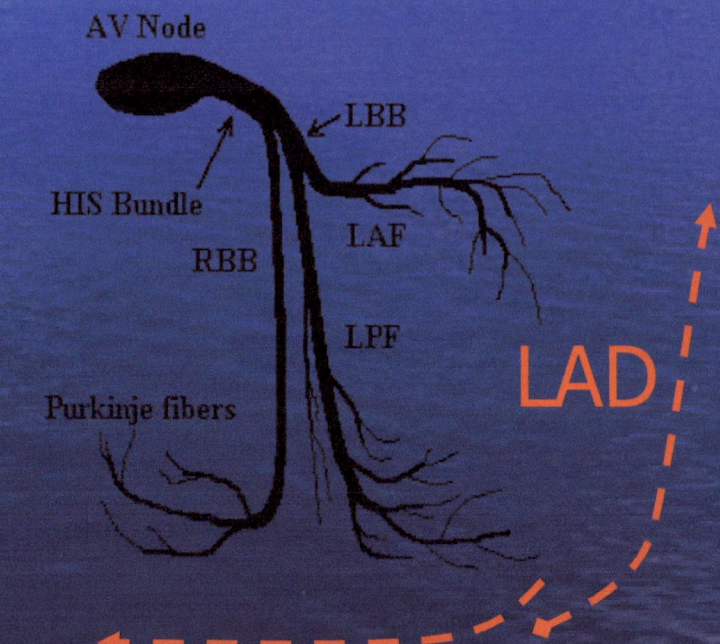

LAD

RAD

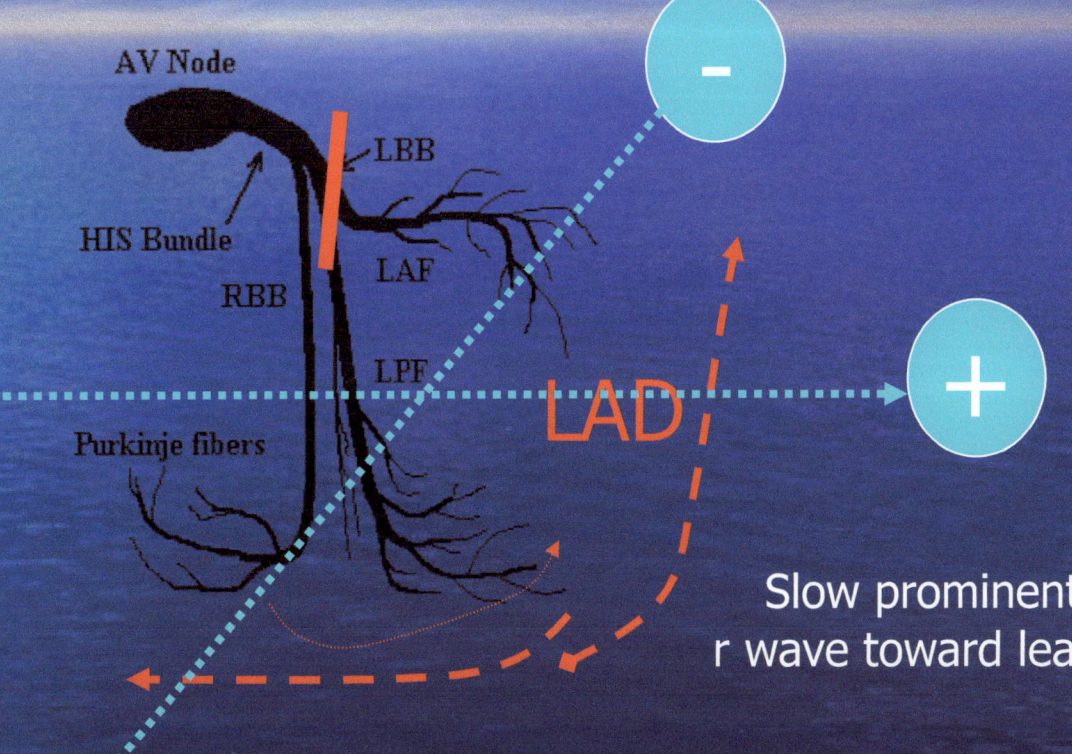

Left Bundle Branch Block

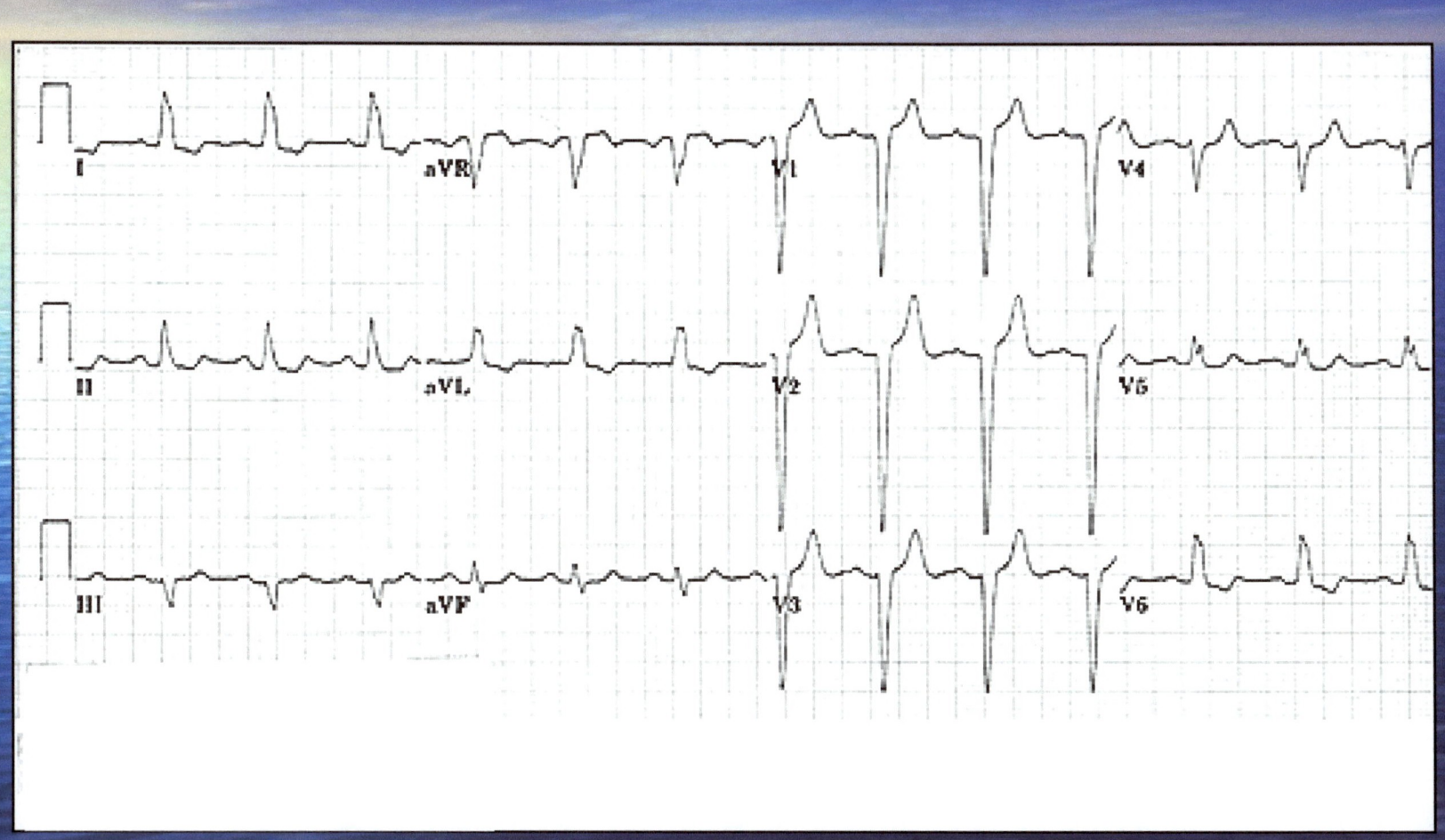

Osborne (J-waves)-Hypothermia

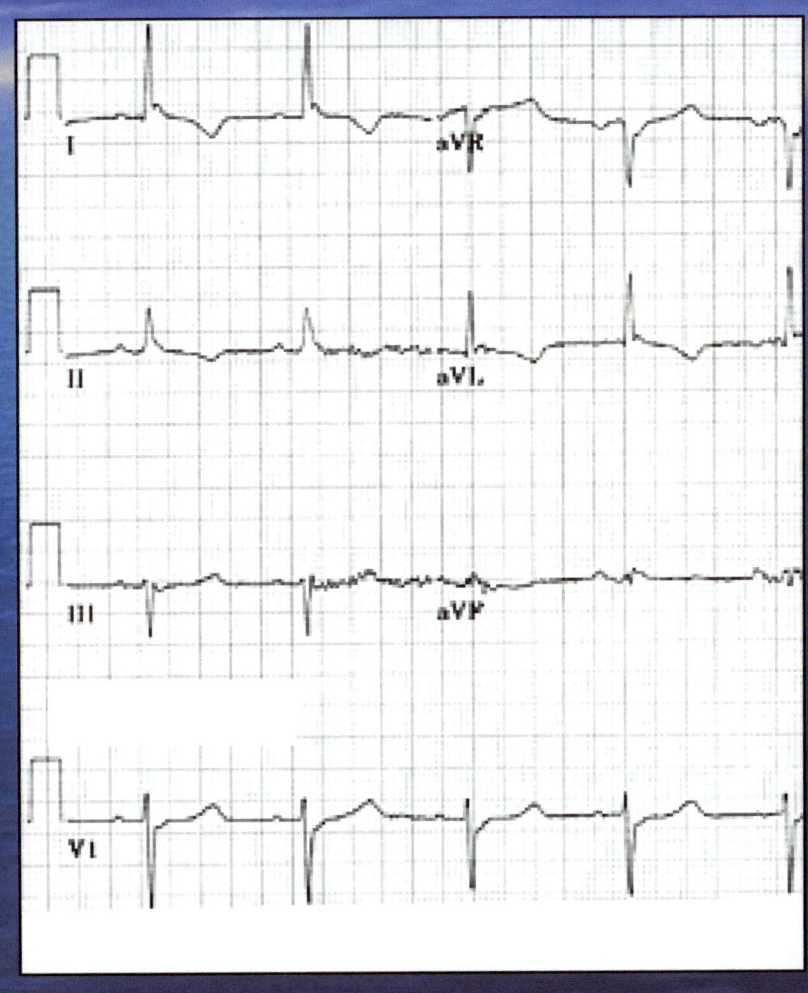

Unique waves with wide QRS

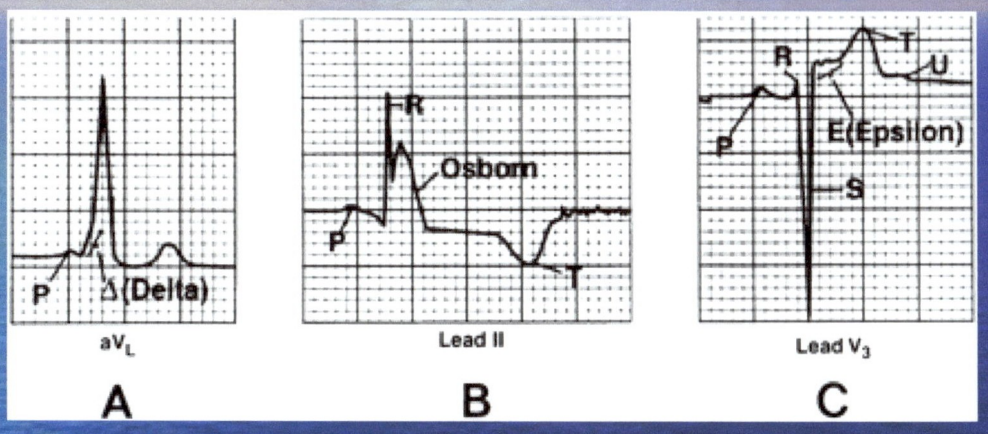

- Delta wave = pre-excitation
- Osborne (J-wave) = wide QRS with spike & dome and prolonged QT = hypothermia, hypercalcemia.
- Epsilon wave = arrythmogenic right ventricular dysplasia

Brugada Syndrome: Wide QRS with ST elevation with 2nd R.

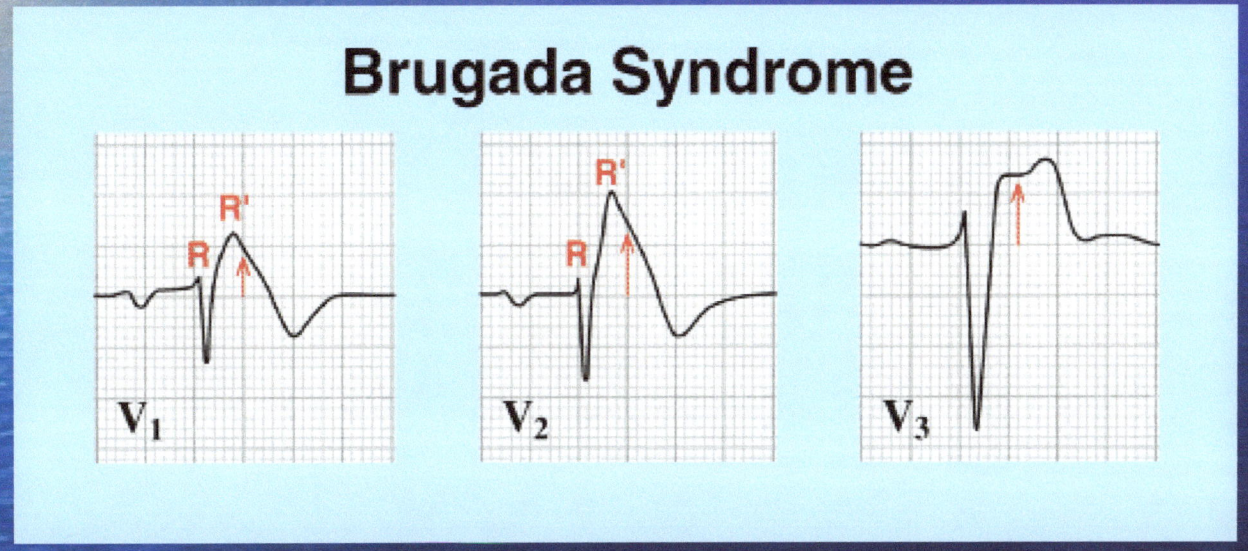

½ of all sudden death, familial malfunction of Na+ channels

Measure the QRS.
What is the Rhythm?

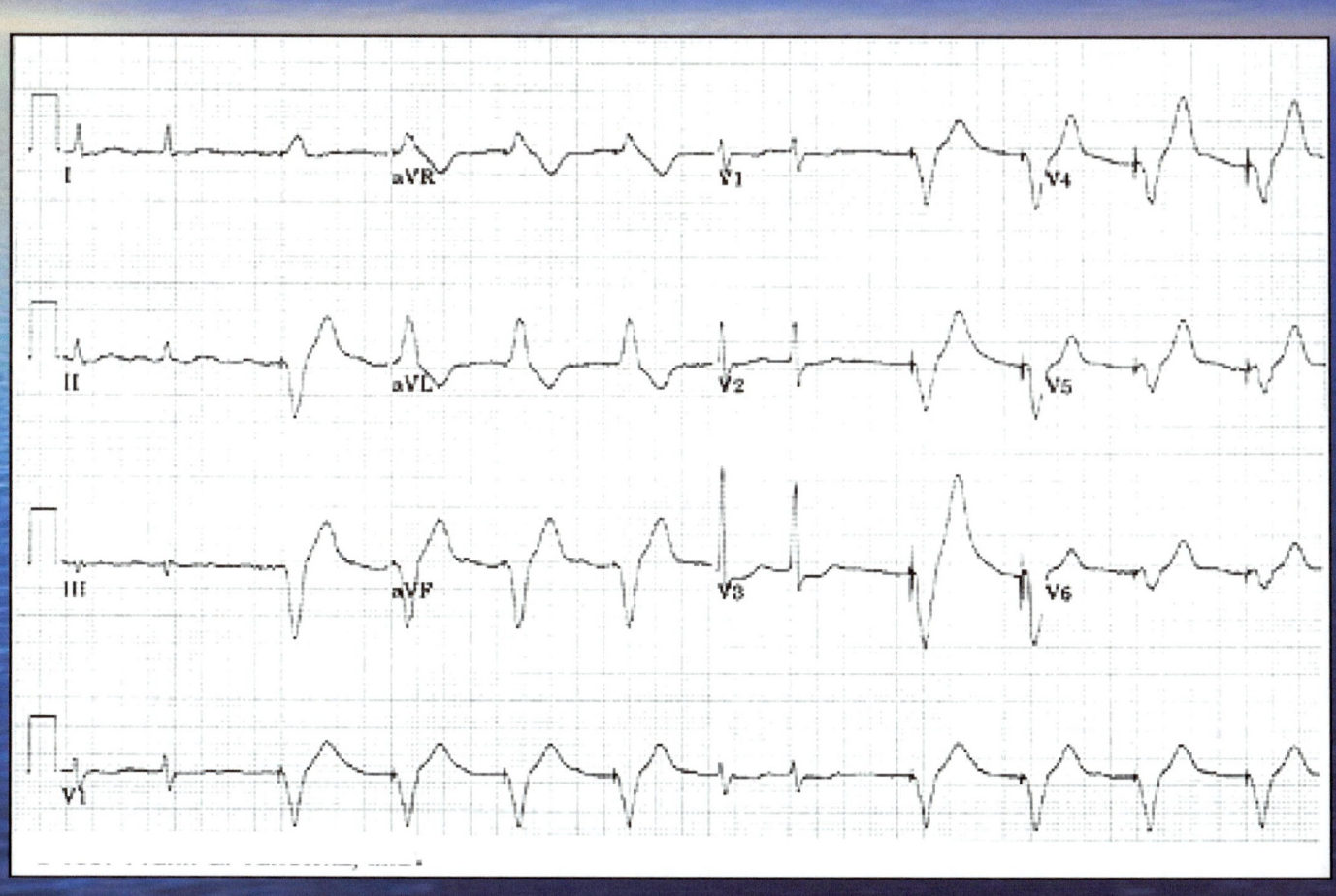

What is the PR Interval?
What is the duration of QRS?

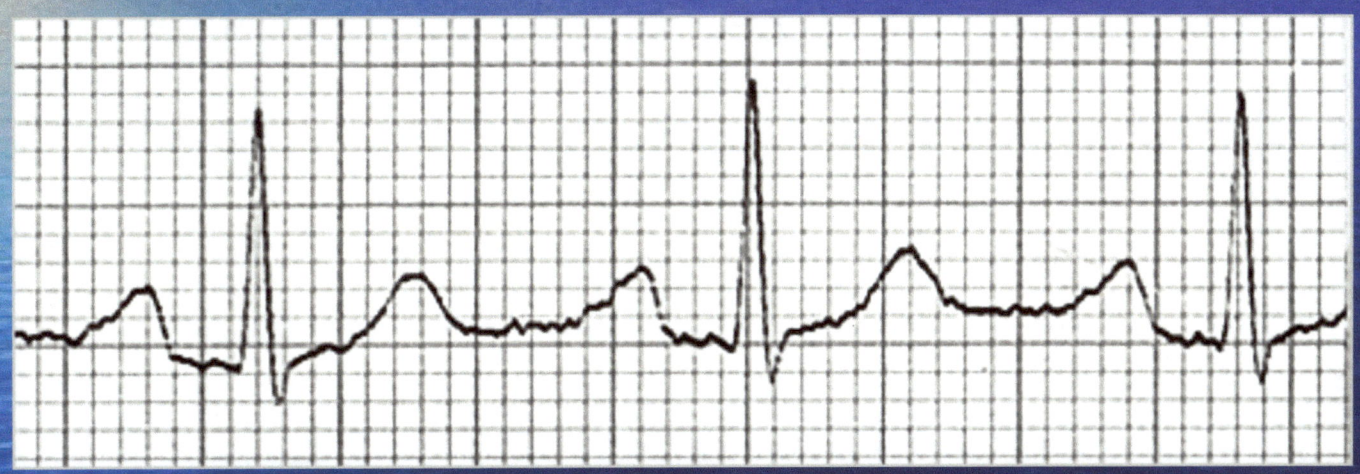

Is the QRS wide and why?

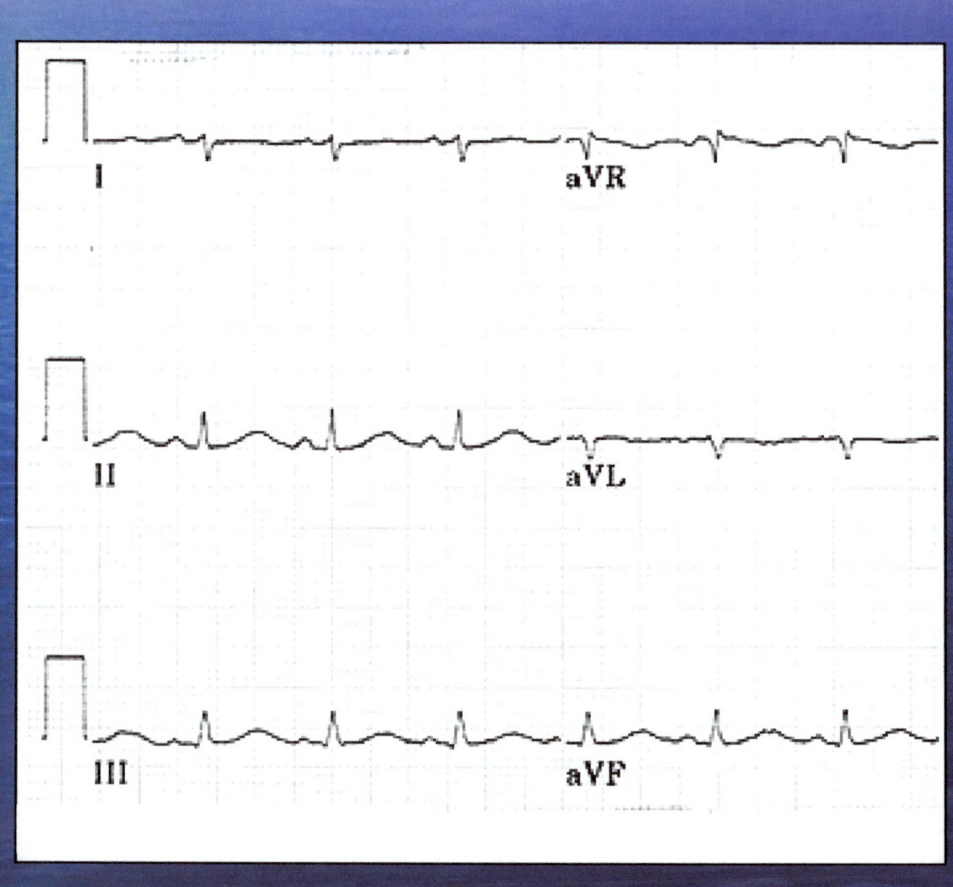

Today & Next Time.

- Today
  - How to determine QRS axis.
  - How to measure QRS length
    - Normal, IVCD including fascicular blocks &
    - Prolonged QRS including bundle branch blocks, pacing and specific wide QRSs that are indicative of accessory pathways, epicardial injury or prorhythmic.
- Next Time
  - ST segments including how to distinguish MIs from other abnormalities
  - T-waves and U-waves.

Normal Electrical Depolarization of the Heart.

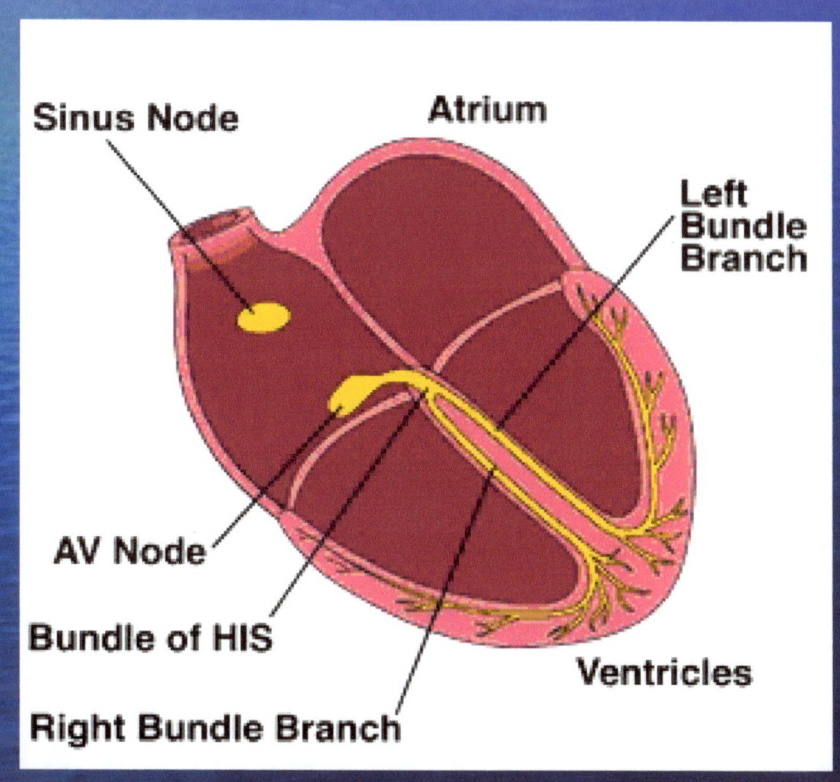

Lecture #3. Ventricular Depolarization & Repolarization: QRS, QT, T & U.

- Matching QRST with the Depolarization and Repolarization of the Ventricles.
- QT interval
  - The movement of cations across cell membranes.
- ST changes
  - Ischemia, infarction, aneurysm, pericarditis.
- T waves
  - The refractory period, all things being relative.
- U waves
  - Repolarization of papillary muscles in bradycardia
  - Or an electrolyte problem?

What are the Names of the Cardiac Pacemaker Cells?

- What is the other name for the Sino-atrial node
  - Keith-Flack's node
  - The left portion is also called the
    - Pace-Bryni-Segre node
- What is the other name for the Atrio-Ventricular node?
  - Tawara-Aschoff's node

Cellular Depolarization (Action Potential) vary from Beginning to End.

Pacemaker Action Potentials (SA & AV) are slow rising, slower and of smaller amplitude.
Non-pacemaker Action Potentials (Atria, AV Bundle, His-Purkinje System & Ventricles) are rapid rising, conduct rapidly and of larger amplitude.

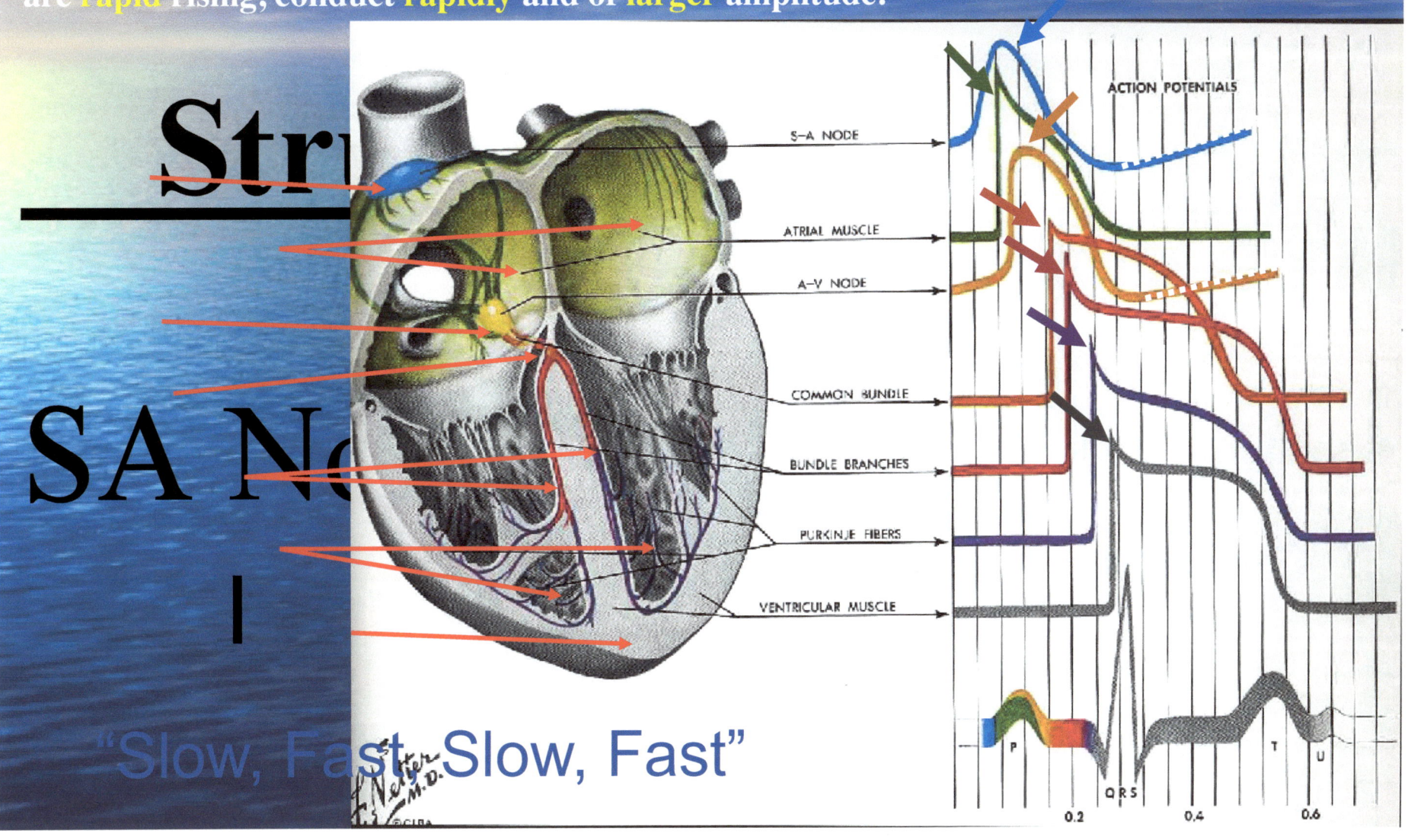

"Slow, Fast, Slow, Fast"

Action Potential of Bundle of His & Myocardium.

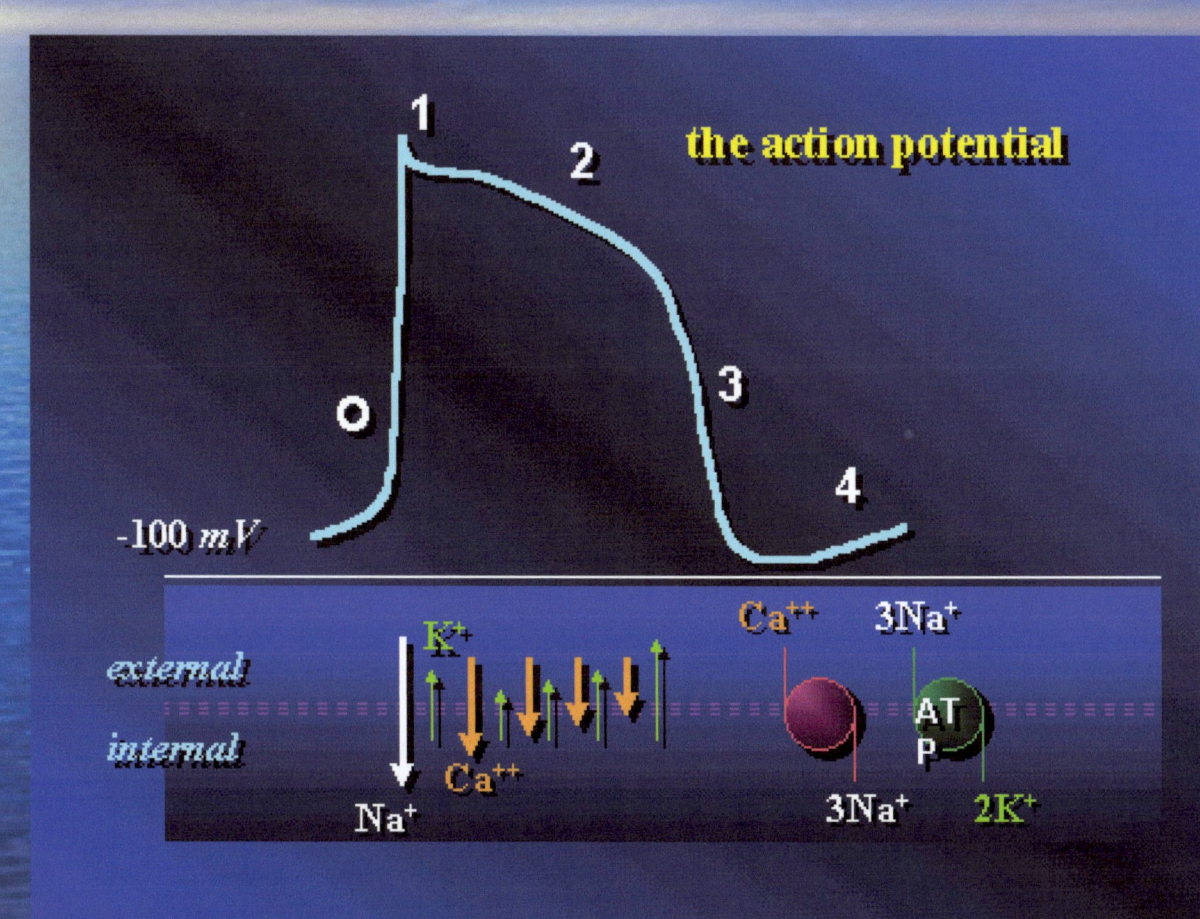

Relationship Between Ventricular Action Potential and the QRS Complex:

Depolarization: Upstrokes (phase 0) of all of the action potentials generated as the wave of depolarization spreads over the ventricles.
The movement of Sodium and the site of action of Class I a,b,& c Drugs.

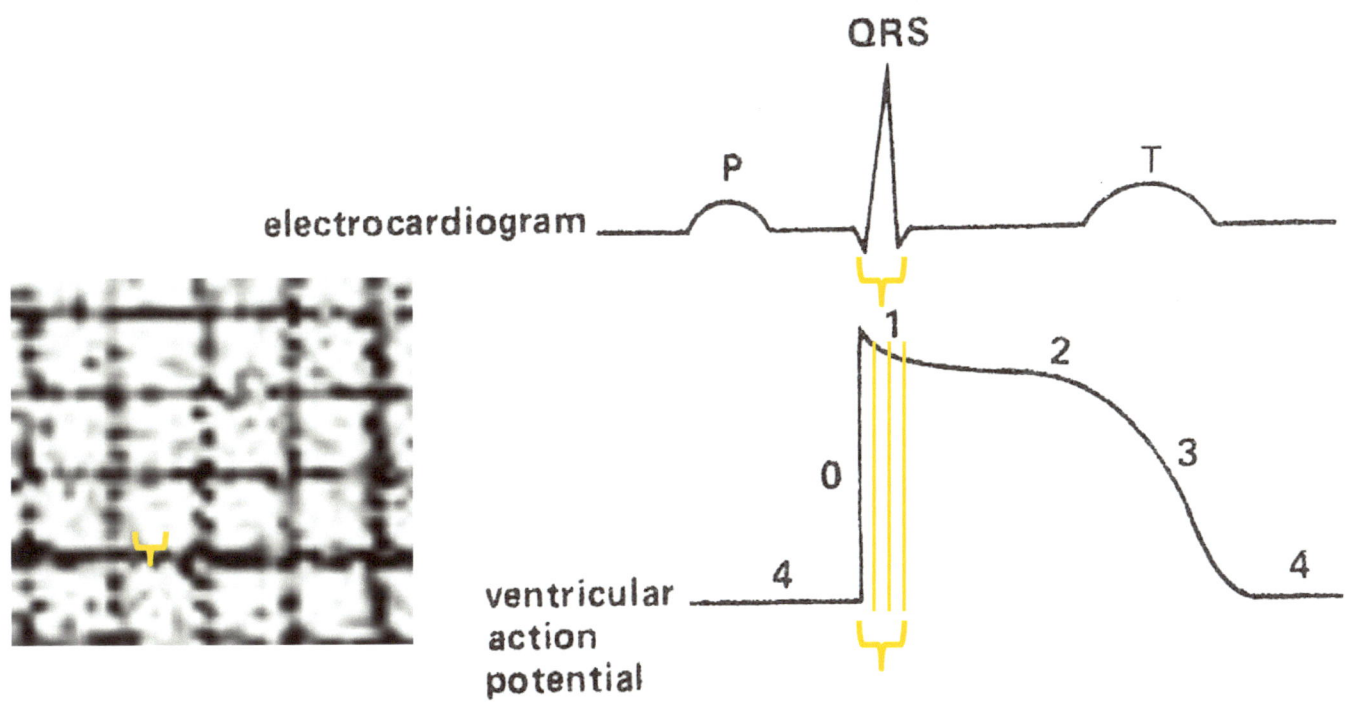

FIG. 20-12. Temporal relationships between the ECG **(top)** and a representative cardiac action potential **(bottom)**. The QRS complex is produced by the upstrokes (phase 0) of all of the action potentials in the ventricles; the isoelectric S–T segment corresponds to the plateau (phase 2), and the T wave is inscribed during repolarization (phase 3) of the ventricular mass. The isoelectric segment that follows the T wave, called the T–P segment, is inscribed during ventricular diastole (phase 4).

Relationship Between Ventricular Action Potential and the ST Segment:
Occurs when all regions of the ventricles are depolarized during the plateau (phase 2) of the cardiac action potential.
The movement of Calcium (& K+) and the site of action of Class III & IV Drugs.

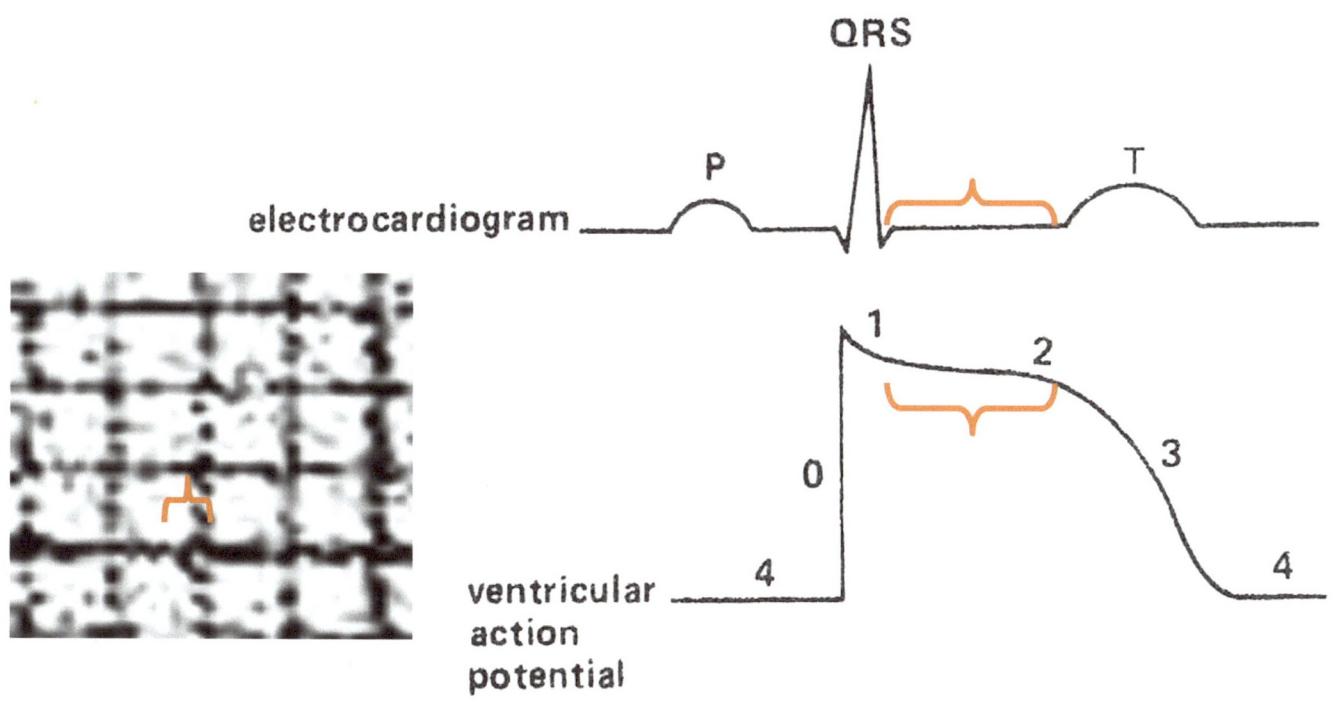

FIG. 20-12. Temporal relationships between the ECG **(top)** and a representative cardiac action potential **(bottom).** The QRS complex is produced by the upstrokes (phase 0) of all of the action potentials in the ventricles; the isoelectric S–T segment corresponds to the plateau (phase 2), and the T wave is inscribed during repolarization (phase 3) of the ventricular mass. The isoelectric segment that follows the T wave, called the T–P segment, is inscribed during ventricular diastole (phase 4).

Relationship Between Ventricular Action Potential and the T wave:

Occurs when all regions of the ventricles are repolarized during phase 3 of the cardiac action potential.

The movement of Potassium and the site of action of Class III Drugs extending the refractory period, blocking re-entrant tachy-dysrhythmias.

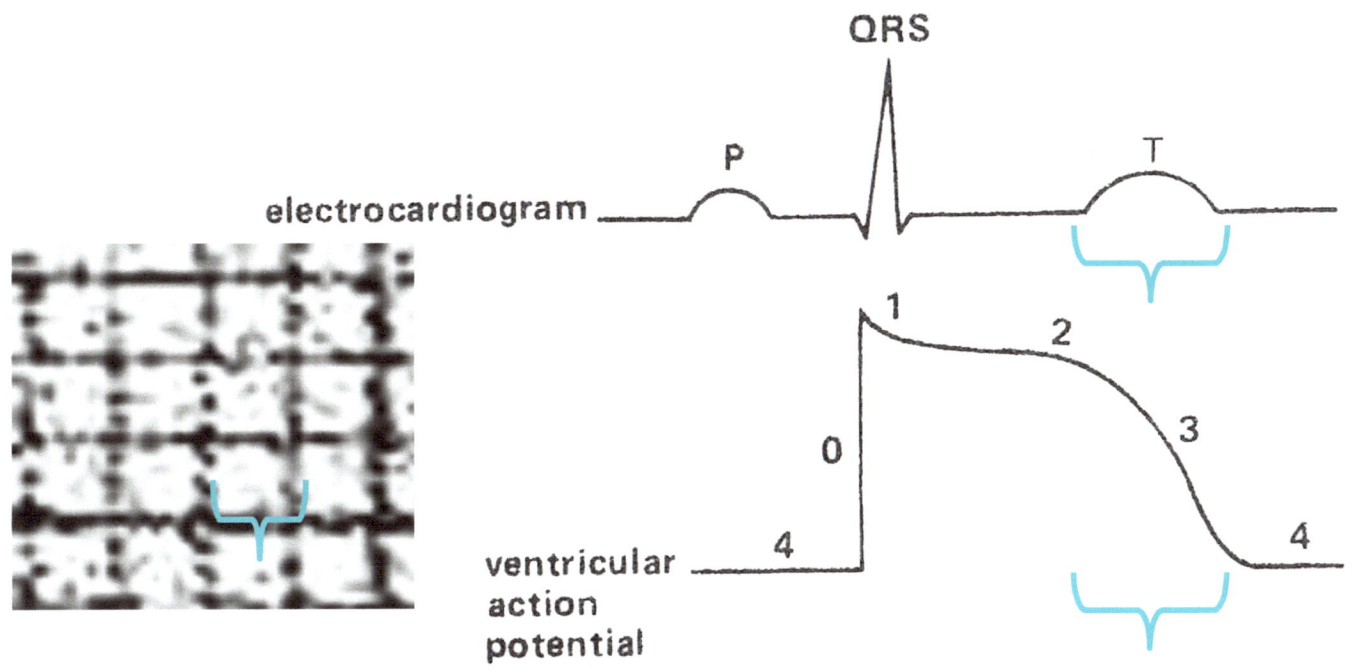

FIG. 20-12. Temporal relationships between the ECG **(top)** and a representative cardiac action potential **(bottom).** The QRS complex is produced by the upstrokes (phase 0) of all of the action potentials in the ventricles; the isoelectric S–T segment corresponds to the plateau (phase 2), and the T wave is inscribed during repolarization (phase 3) of the ventricular mass. The isoelectric segment that follows the T wave, called the T–P segment, is inscribed during ventricular diastole (phase 4).

Relationship Between Ventricular Action Potential and the TP Interval:
Occurs during ventricular diastole.
The movement of Sodium and Potassium and the site of action of Class II Drugs.

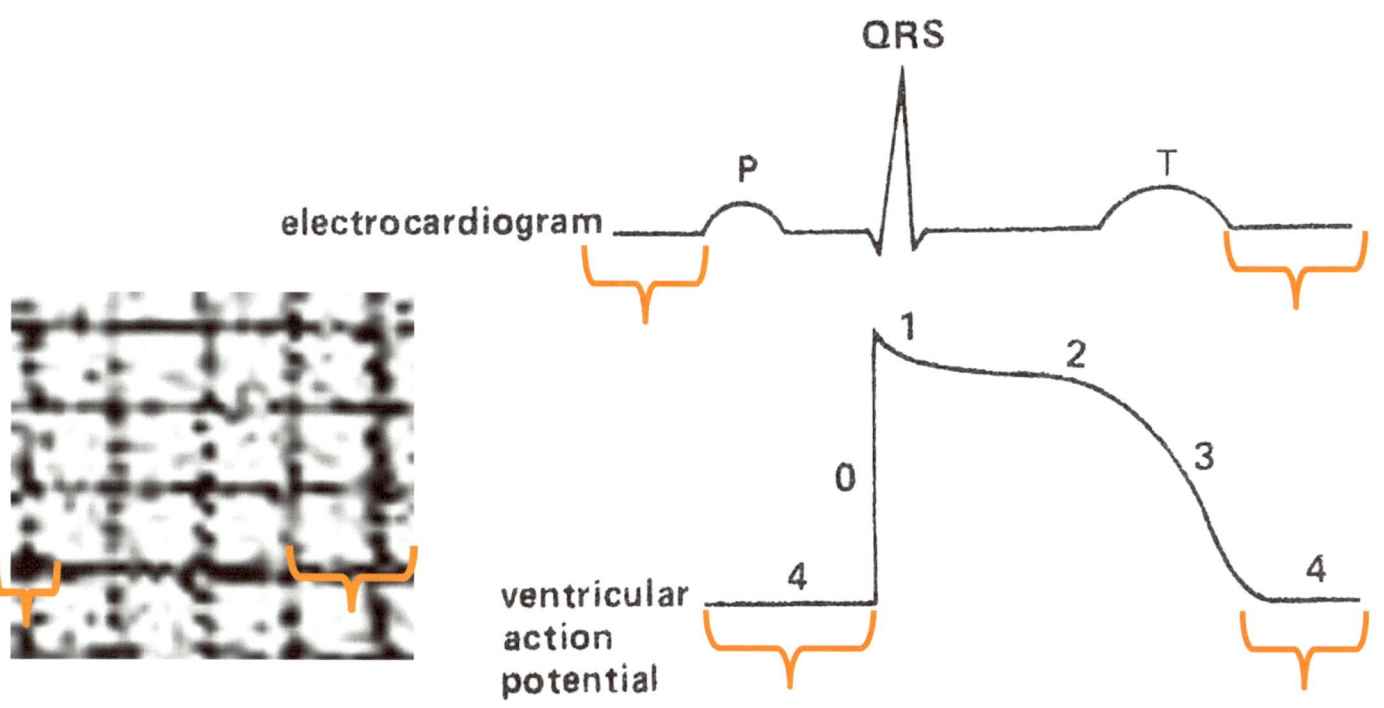

FIG. 20-12. Temporal relationships between the ECG **(top)** and a representative cardiac action potential **(bottom)**. The QRS complex is produced by the upstrokes (phase 0) of all of the action potentials in the ventricles; the isoelectric S–T segment corresponds to the plateau (phase 2), and the T wave is inscribed during repolarization (phase 3) of the ventricular mass. The isoelectric segment that follows the T wave, called the T–P segment, is inscribed during ventricular diastole (phase 4).

Relationship Between Ventricular Action Potential and the ECG QT Interval:
An overall index of the duration of the ventricular action potential. Anything affecting these changes can affect ventricular depolarization & the QT interval.

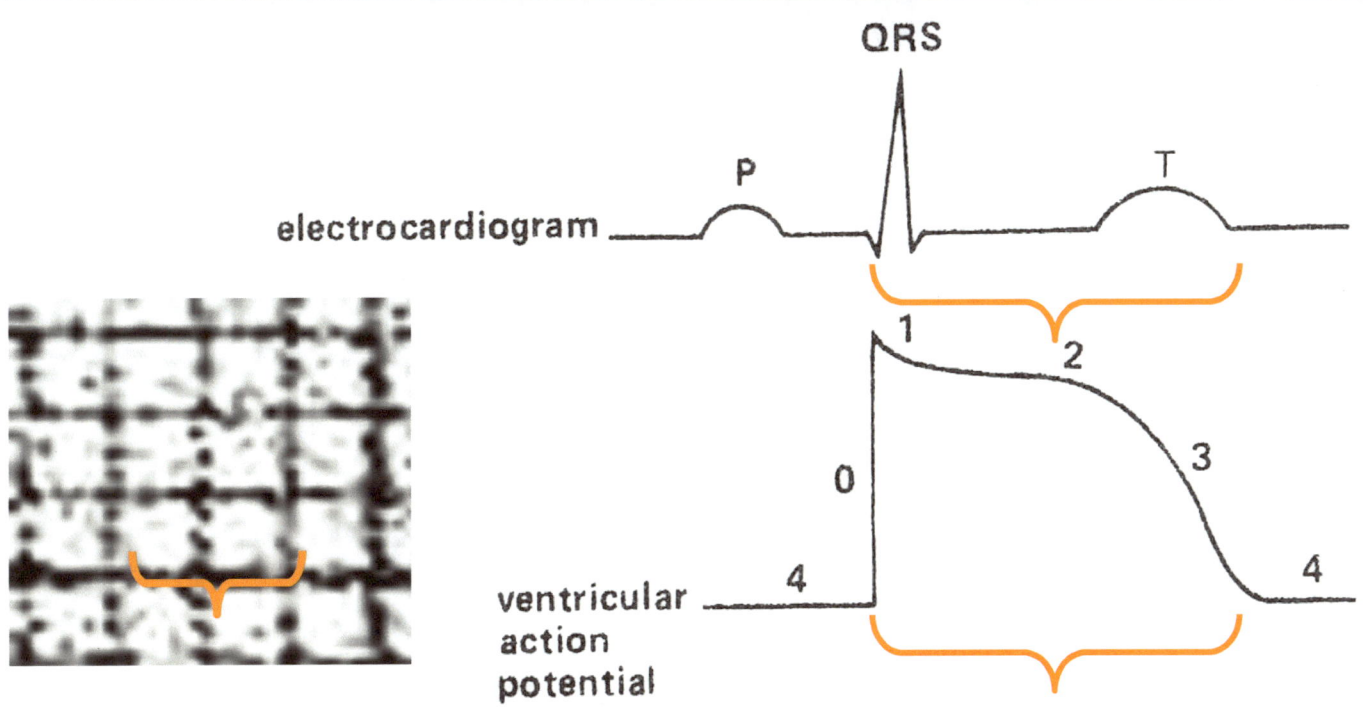

FIG. 20-12. Temporal relationships between the ECG **(top)** and a representative cardiac action potential **(bottom)**. The QRS complex is produced by the upstrokes (phase 0) of all of the action potentials in the ventricles; the isoelectric S–T segment corresponds to the plateau (phase 2), and the T wave is inscribed during repolarization (phase 3) of the ventricular mass. The isoelectric segment that follows the T wave, called the T–P segment, is inscribed during ventricular diastole (phase 4).

The QT Interval

- QT is the measurement from beginning of Q-wave to end of T-wave
  - However, the depolarization and repolarization time varies depending upon HR.
  - The faster the HR, the more rapid the movement of cations across the membranes.
    - Shortening the QT interval.
  - The opposite is true for slowing of HR.
- Corrected QT (QTc) takes into account these changes in QT resulting from changes in HR.
  - QTc = measured QT/sq-root RR in seconds
    - upper limit for QT**c** $\sim$ 44% of the RR interval

Measuring the QT Interval.
The amount of time it takes the ventricles to depolarize and repolarize in preparation for the next electrical (hopefully atrial) impulse.

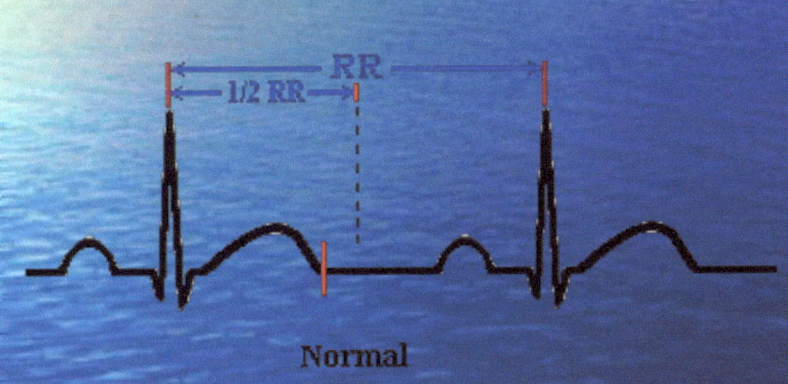

Normal

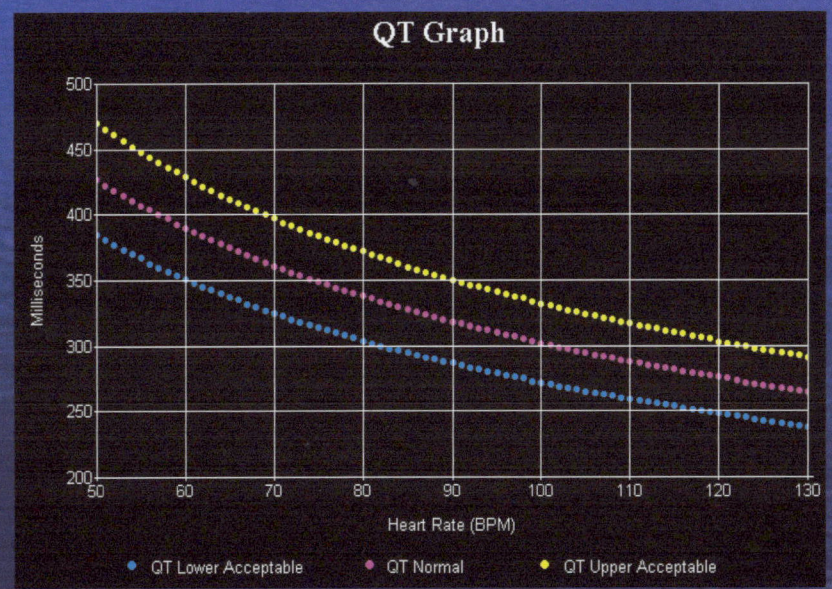

Bazett's Formula:

$$QTc = \sqrt{\frac{QT\ measured}{RR\ \text{(in seconds)}}}$$

Normal QTc

0.39 ♂   0.41 ♀

The QT Interval (cont):

- Long QT syndrome (LQTS)
  - In men (>0.47 sec or 470 mSec)
  - In women (>0.48 sec or 480 mSec)
- A prolonged QT increases the vulnerability of the ventricles to a malignant ventricular dysrhythmia.
  - Eg. polymorphic VT (viz. Torsade-de-Pointes)
- Short QT Interval
  - Defined as < 0.30 sec
    - Familial tendency for increased ventricular fibrillation*
  - Like most things, too much or too little of something can produce problems.

* Circulation 2003;108:965

Causes of Prolonged QT.

- In medicine you must ask more than what do I see, you must ask why am I seeing it?
- Causes:
  - Drugs (many antiarrhythmics [eg. Ia], tricyclics, phenothiazines, and others)
    - Over 200 medications lengthen the QRS.
  - Electrolyte abnormalities
    - Hypokalemia, hypocalcemia, hypomagnesemia
  - CNS disease (especially subarrachnoid hemorrhage, stroke, trauma)
    - Primarily NSST changes and inverted T-waves
  - Hereditary LQTS (e.g., Romano-Ward Syndrome)
  - Coronary Heart Disease (some post-MI patients)

The Effect of Cardiac Drugs on Cellular Depolarization (viz. QT).

- **Class I:** block sodium channels
  - Ia (quinidine, procainamide, disopyramide) ↑AP
  - Ib (lidocaine) ↓AP
  - Ic (flecainide) ↔AP
- **Class II:** ß-adrenoceptor antagonists (atenolol, sotalol)
- **Class III:** prolong action potential and prolong refractory period (suppress re-entrant rhythms) (amiodarone, sotalol)
- **Class IV:** Calcium channel antagonists. Impair impulse propagation in nodal and damaged areas (verapamil)

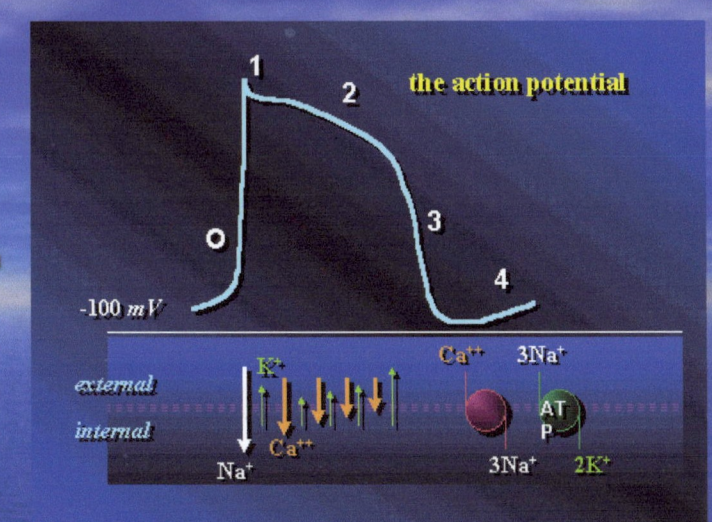
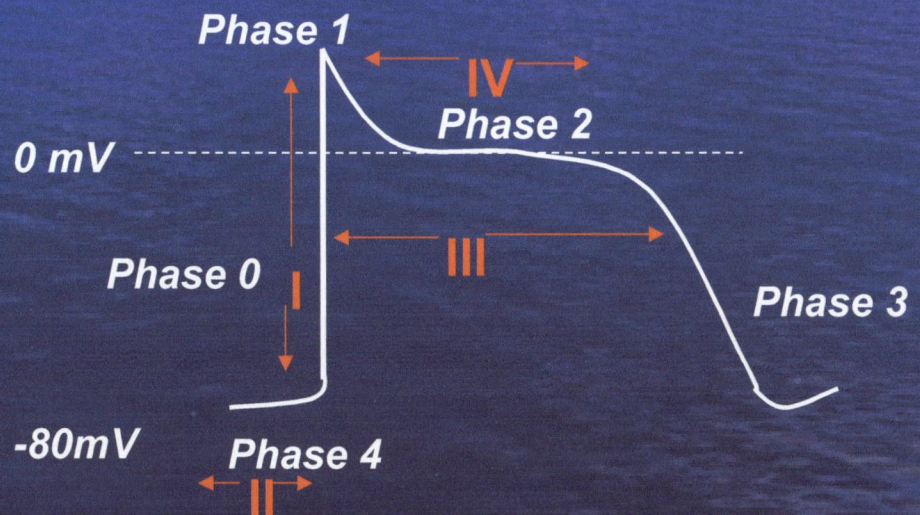

Changes in Calcium Change QT.

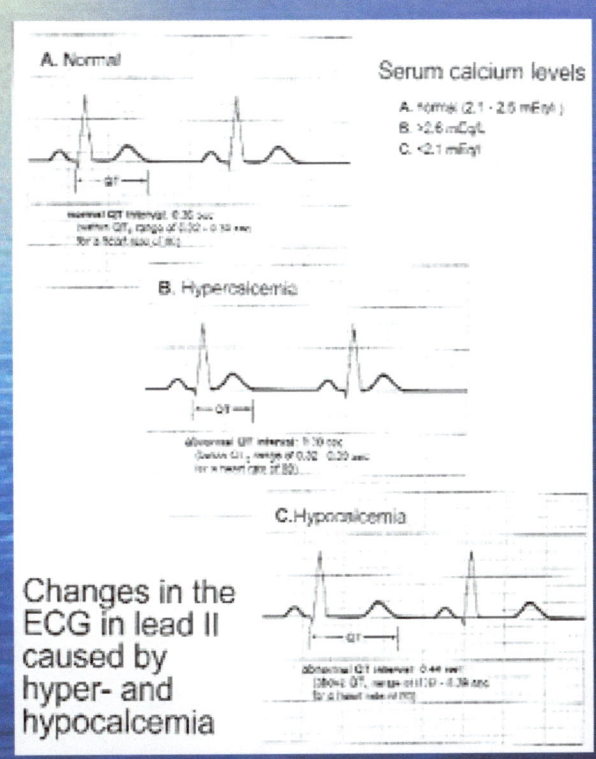

Changes in the ECG in lead II caused by hyper- and hypocalcemia

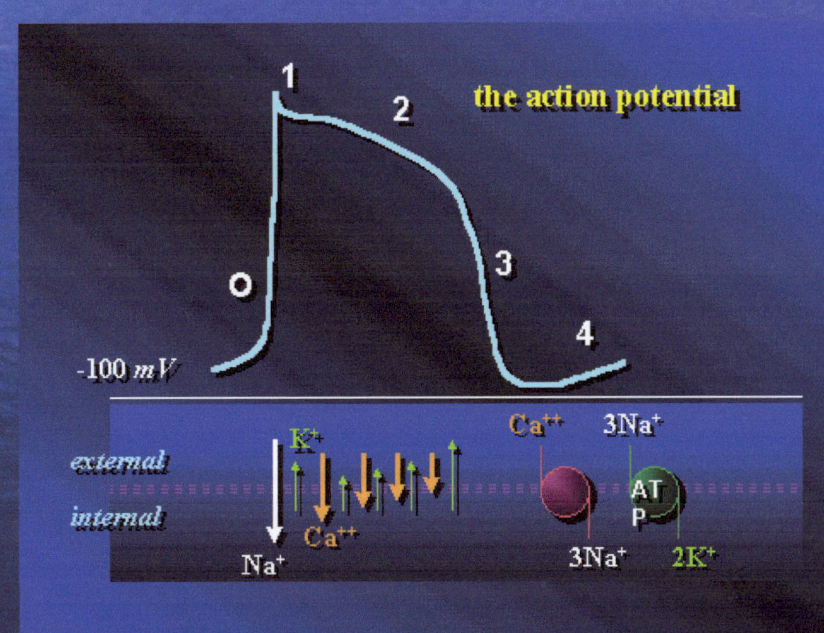

the action potential

Hypocalcemia and the QT.

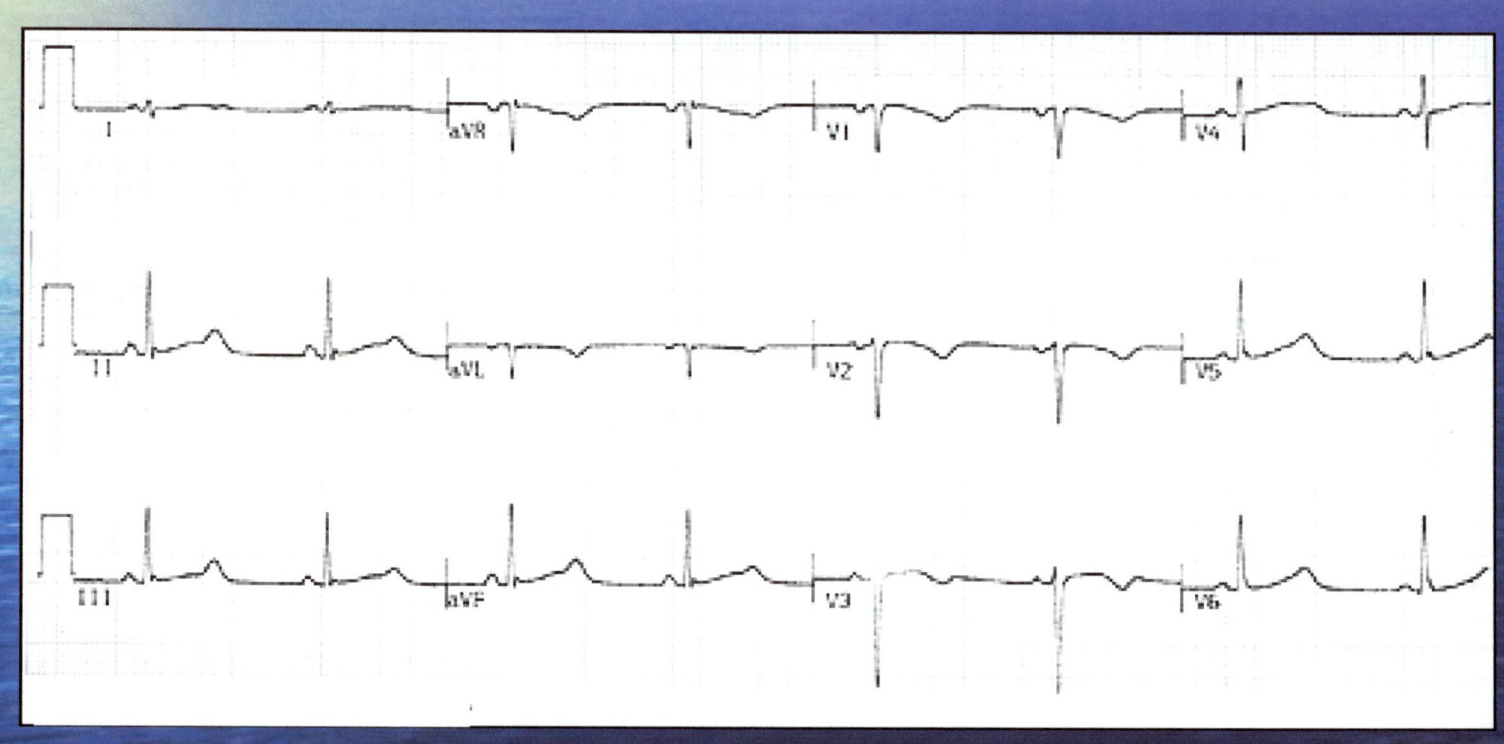

Subarrachnoid hemorrhage

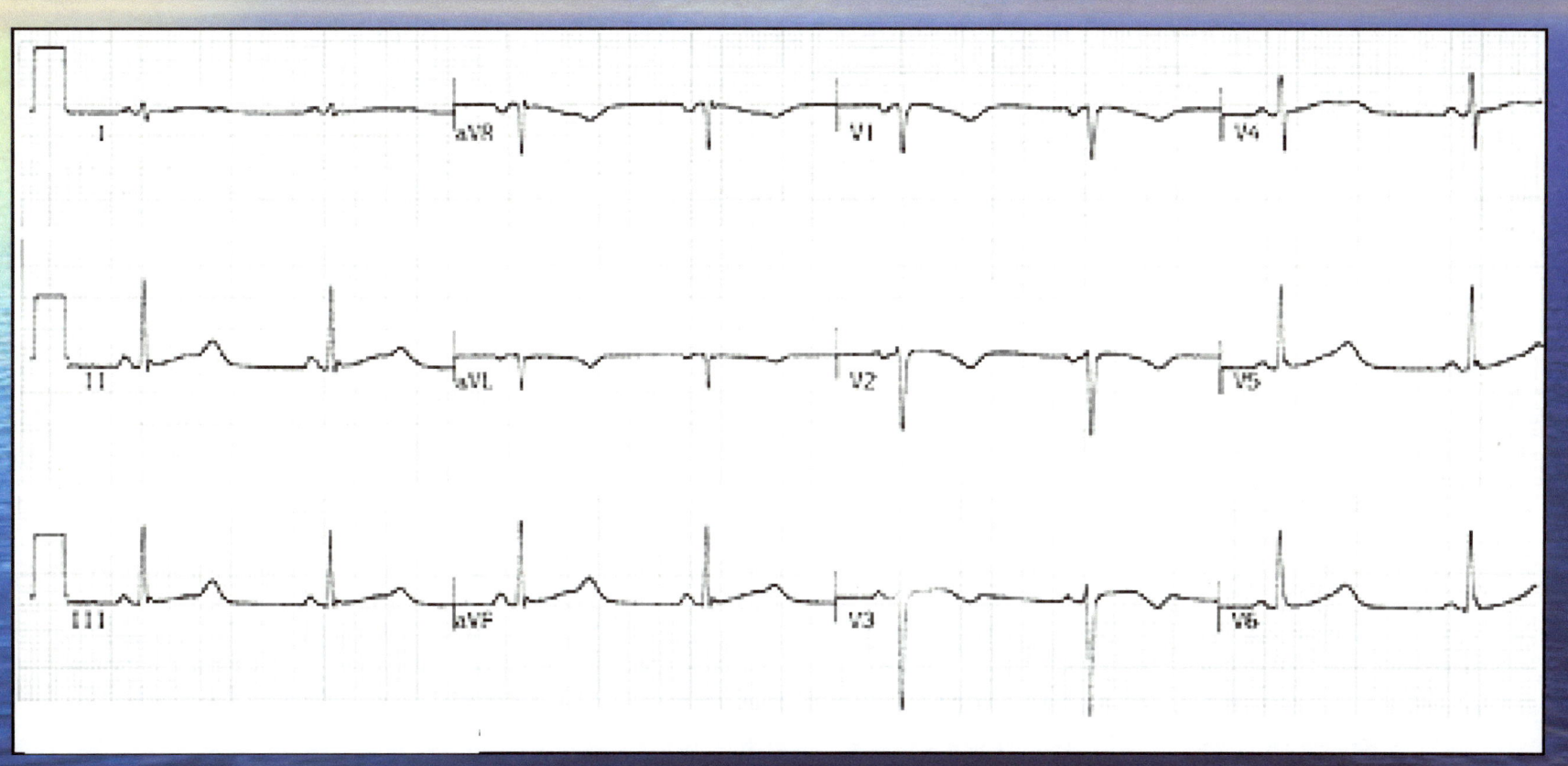

Romano-Ward Syndrome

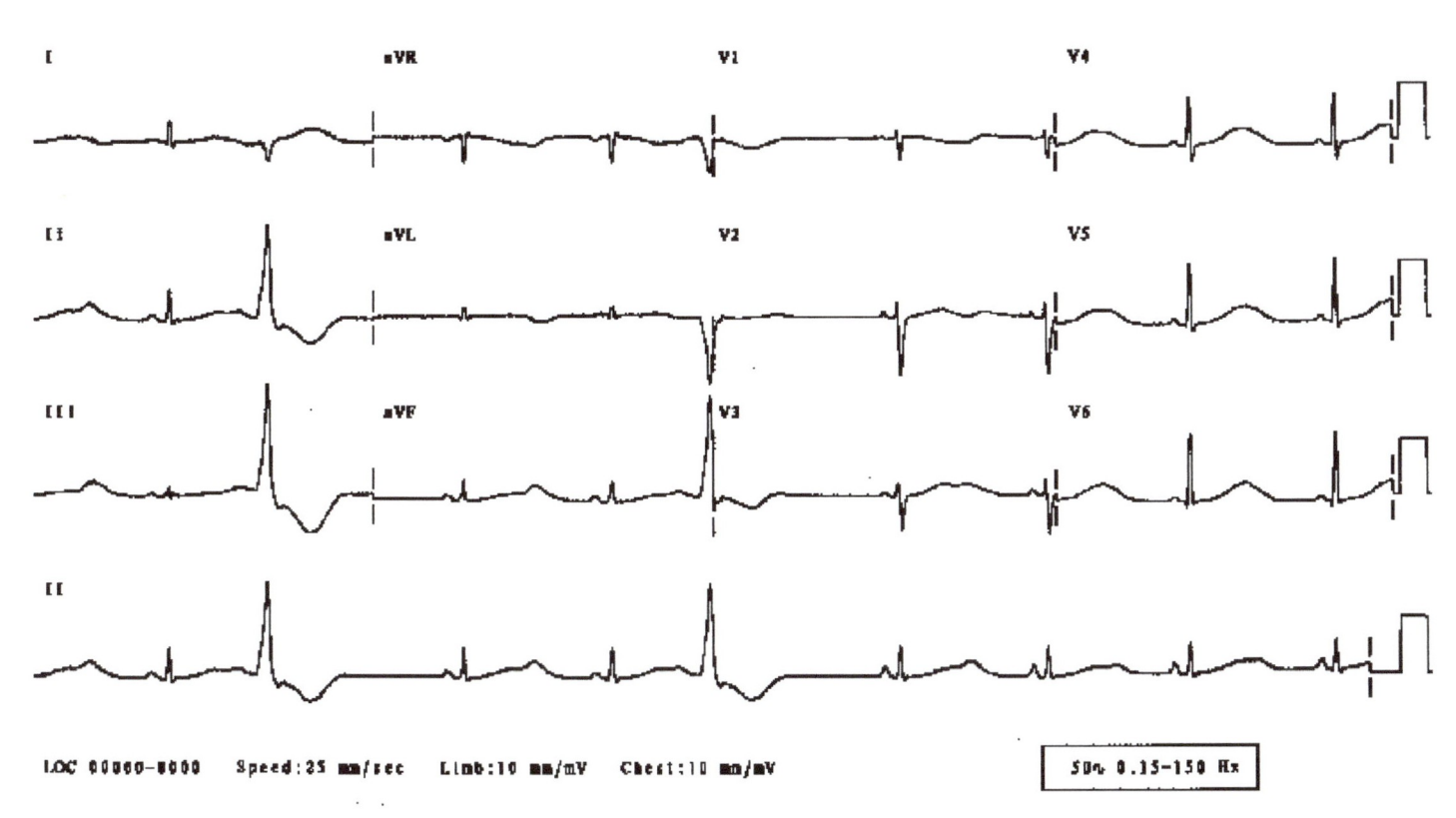

Short QT Interval

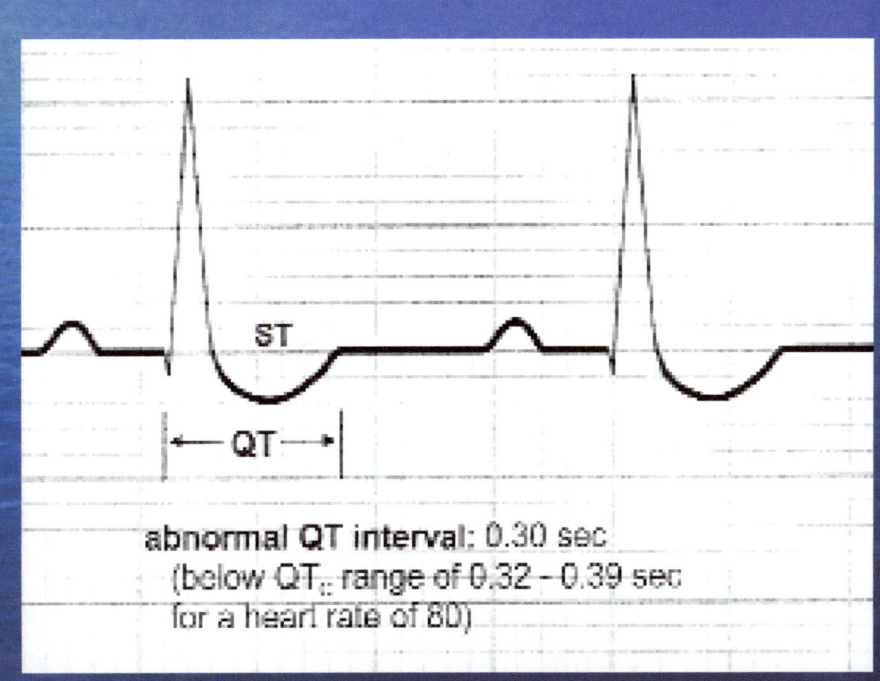

What is the QT Interval?

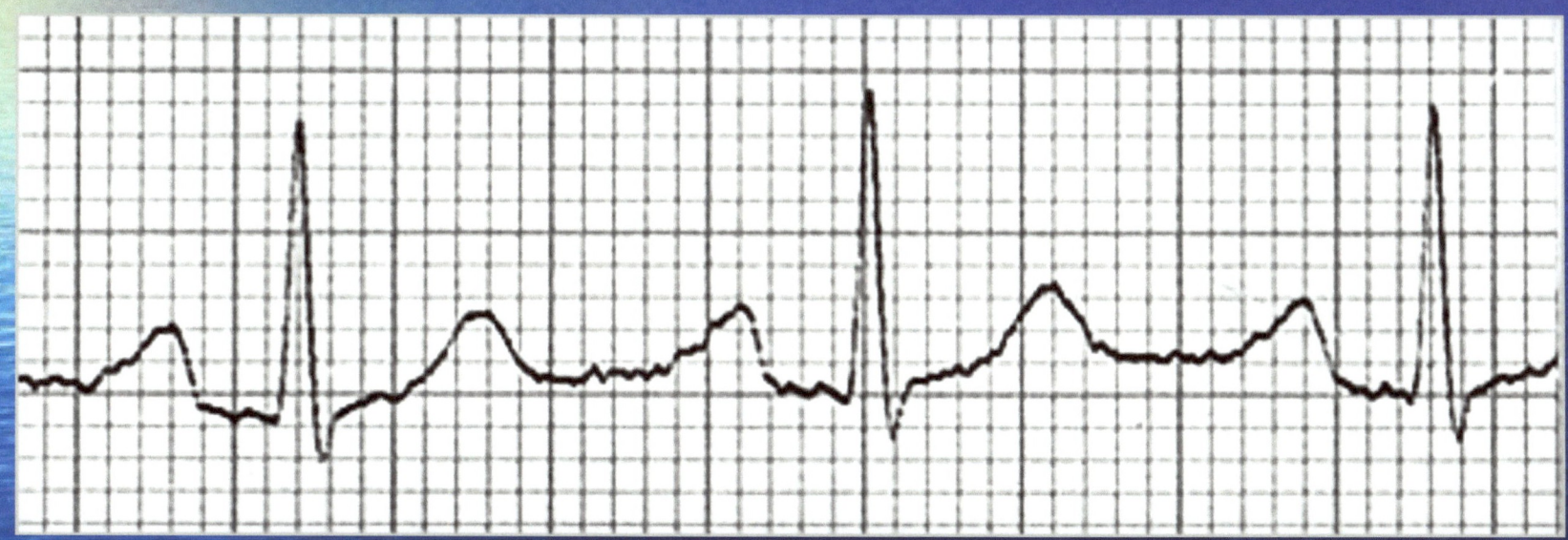

Measuring the QT Interval.
Name 3 possible causes for this ECG.

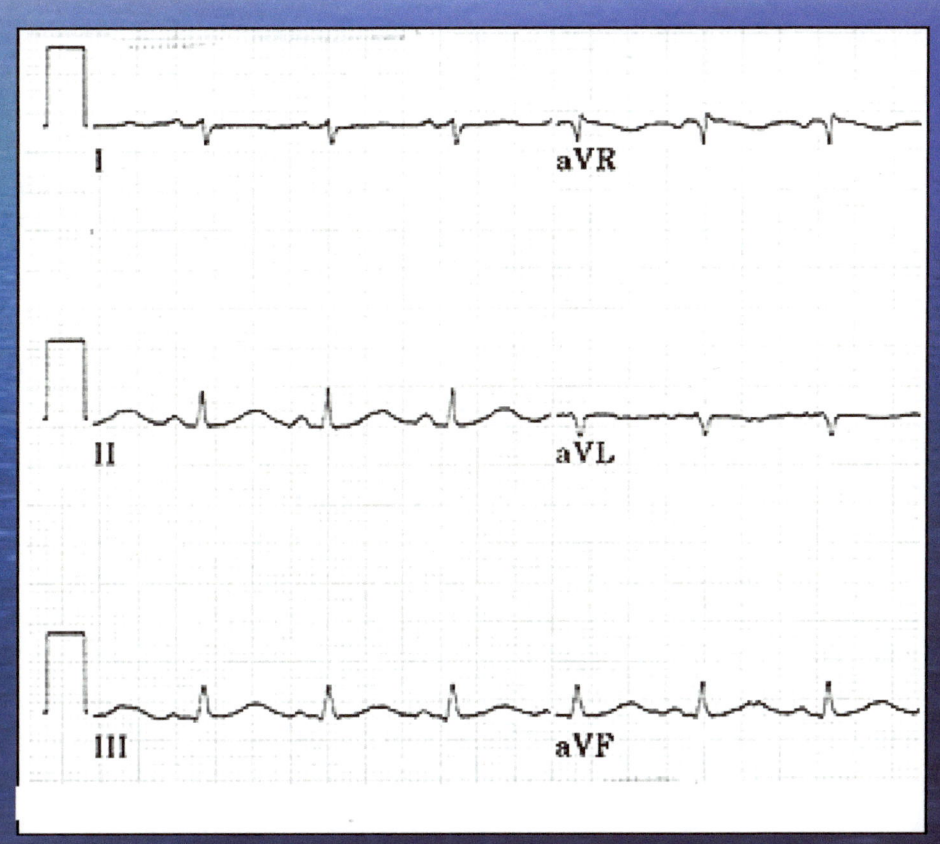

In the next series of slides we will begin with changes in the ST segment and learn how to interpret myocardial ischemia and infarction.

www.ingramcontent.com/pod-product-compliance
Lightning Source LLC
Chambersburg PA
CBHW051154220526
45473CB00003B/769